Societies are lively, dynamic and made and re-made through social practices that involve microbial lives. Insightful and innovative, and providing glimpses of a better future, the interdisciplinary authors take social practices and microbial relations as fundamental to understanding planetary wellbeing, health and welfare.

Steve Hinchliffe, *Chair in Environmental Geography, School of Geography, University of Oxford*

Social Practices and Microscopic Matter lays the foundation for critical scholarship on human-microbial relations. An important text for all interested in micro-ecological stewardship and creating 'probiotic' communities in a time of global pandemics and antimicrobial resistance.

Rachael Wakefield-Rann, *Research Principal, Institute for Sustainable Futures, University of Technology Sydney*

SOCIAL PRACTICES AND MICROSCOPIC MATTER

It is widely recognised that biological, microbial and social processes constitute each other, but there is much less agreement about what this means, or about how this interweaving should be conceptualised and studied. Whilst recognising that there has been huge growth in more-than-human approaches and in contributions from science and technology studies and feminist scholarship, this volume advocates that more ideas are needed if we are to address global threats, including the impacts of climate change, growing antimicrobial resistance, pandemics, the geographies and distribution of zoonoses and other large biosocial phenomena.

Contributors from disciplines including anthropology, geography, sociology and public health bring these resources to bear on fundamental questions about scale and transmission, the place of human bodies in social and biological theory, and concepts of health, risk and disease. Informed by real-life examples relating to food, insects, water and air, the spread of disease and antimicrobial resistance, the result is an agenda-setting book positioned at the intersection of research and policy.

It will appeal to scholars and academics with interest in social theory, microbes and public health, as well as academics and advanced students of geography, anthropology, sociology, medical sociology, social studies of science and the history of health.

Elizabeth Shove is Emeritus Professor of Sociology at Lancaster University. She is well known for her work on social theories of practice.

Cecily Maller is Professor of Human Geography at the Centre for Urban Research, School of Global, Urban and Social Studies, RMIT University, Australia. She is interested in human-environment relationships in urban settings and their implications for health outcomes.

Simon Cohn is Professor in Medical Anthropology at the London School of Hygiene and Tropical Medicine, United Kingdom. Simon is a medical anthropologist with a particular interest in biomedicine and public health in the UK and other high-income settings.

SOCIAL PRACTICES AND MICROSCOPIC MATTER

Challenging Ideas about Bodies, Microbes and Health

Edited by Elizabeth Shove, Cecily Maller and Simon Cohn

Routledge
Taylor & Francis Group
LONDON AND NEW YORK

Designed cover image: Elizabeth Shove

First published 2027
by Routledge
4 Park Square, Milton Park, Abingdon, Oxon OX14 4RN

and by Routledge
605 Third Avenue, New York, NY 10158

Routledge is an imprint of the Taylor & Francis Group, an informa business

British Library Cataloguing-in-Publication Data
A catalogue record for this book is available from the British Library

ISBN: 9781041165583 (hbk)
ISBN: 9781041165569 (pbk)
ISBN: 9781003685210 (ebk)

DOI: 10.4324/9781003685210

Typeset in Sabon
by Newgen Publishing UK

CONTENTS

CONTRIBUTORS

Stanley Blue, Department of Sociology, Lancaster University, Lancaster, United Kingdom. Stanley is author of *Practice Theory and Process Philosophy: Towards a Sociology of Becoming* (Routledge, 2025), and editor of the *Journal of Practice Theory*.

Karl Broome, Department of Political and Social Sciences, Universitat Pompeu Fabra, Spain. Karl's PhD research deals with exposure to mosquito-borne disease and tourist practices in Barcelona.

Nik Brown, Department of Sociology, University of York, United Kingdom. Nik, who is Professor and Head of Department, writes extensively about the sociology of health and the body focusing particularly on the biopolitics of immunity.

Christina Buse, Department of Sociology, University of York, United Kingdom. Christina is a Lecturer in Sociology and has used creative methods to explore experiences of dementia, health and illness, ageing, place and material culture.

Simon Cohn, London School of Hygiene and Tropical Medicine, United Kingdom. Simon is a medical anthropologist with a particular interest in biomedicine and public health in the UK and other high-income settings.

George Cusworth, Department of Philosophy, Classics, History of Art and Ideas, University of Oslo, Norway. George is a Post-Doctoral Researcher whose research focuses on food and agriculture and draws on concepts from geography, political ecology and science and technology studies.

Beth Greenhough, School of Geography and the Environment, University of Oxford, United Kingdom. Beth is a Professor of Human Geography who uses political-economic geography, cultural geography and science studies to explore the social implications of scientific innovations in the areas of health, biomedicine and the environment.

Mikko Jauho, Consumer Society Research Centre, Faculty of Social Sciences, University of Helsinki, Finland. Mikko is a Senior Researcher and founding member of the Centre for the Social Studies of Microbes at the Faculty of Social Sciences, University of Helsinki.

Michael P. Kelly, Primary Care Unit, Department of Public Health and Primary Care, University of Cambridge, United Kingdom. Mike is Professor and Senior Visiting Fellow in the Department of Public Health and Primary Care at Cambridge University.

Jamie Lorimer, School of Geography and the Environment, University of Oxford, United Kingdom. Jamie is a Professor of Environmental Geography who focuses on understandings of nature and their consequences for human and nonhuman life across different spatial scales.

Cecily Maller, Centre for Urban Research, School of Global, Urban and Social Studies, RMIT University, Australia. Cecily is Professor of Human Geography, interested in human-environment relationships in urban settings and their implications for health outcomes.

Daryl Martin, Department of Sociology, Maynooth University, Ireland. Daryl is a Lecturer in Sociology and has written extensively on the sociological aspects of the built environment, with particular interests in architectural design, landscape and urban development.

Maurizio Meloni, School of Humanities and Social Sciences, Deakin University, Australia. Maurizio is a social theorist and a science and technology studies scholar with strong affiliations to the history and philosophy of biology and the health sciences.

Sarah Nettleton, Department of Sociology, University of York, United Kingdom. Sarah is Emerita Professor of Sociology and has written extensively on the sociology of health and illness, the body and embodiment.

Elizabeth Shove, Department of Sociology, Lancaster University, Lancaster, United Kingdom. Elizabeth is Emeritus Professor of Sociology and is well known for her work on social theories of practice.

ACKNOWLEDGEMENTS

Elizabeth Shove, Cecily Maller and Simon Cohn would like to thank the British Academy and Wellcome for supporting the conference, 'Social practice theory and public health: microbes, bodies and environments', June 2025, on which this book is based.

1

SETTING THE SCENE

Conceptualising microbes, bodies and health – Contributions and propositions from social theory

Elizabeth Shove, Cecily Maller and Simon Cohn

Introduction

Like all edited collections, the origins and ambitions of this book are important for the debates with which we engage and the contributions we make. This opening chapter describes how *Social practices and microscopic matter: Challenging ideas about bodies, microbes and health* came about, and what authors draw from, and add to, disciplines as diverse as those of public health, history, geography, sociology and anthropology.

In assembling this volume and in doing so now, we add to a rising tide of interest in the inclusion of microbial life in the social sciences: a tide that is, in turn, linked to increasing concern about the environment in the Anthropocene, and to the popularity of concepts like One Health and Planetary Health. For these reasons and more, it is widely recognised that biological, microbial and social processes constitute each other and that societies are not made by people alone.

That said, there is much less agreement about what this really means and how the interweaving of humans and more-than-humans (living and inert) should be conceptualised and studied. To date, researchers interested in these two-way intra-actions have tended to rely on a narrow band of theoretical resources, often informed by actor network theory or by feminist authors (Barad, 2003; Barad, 2007; Haraway, 2008). Related debates consequently focus on matters of methodological symmetry, the construction of knowledge or the ethics of care (Brives et al., 2021; Cañada et al., 2022).

This collection is inspired by the hunch that there is more to say and that social theories, and theories of practice, in particular, provide a cornucopia of concepts that have yet to be exploited. By dipping into these resources, the

DOI: 10.4324/9781003685210-1

chapters that come next generate new lines of enquiry and reframe questions about contagion, materiality, the boundaries of the body (human and more-than-human), and the part that (human) discourses play in policy and in everyday life. These are powerful and useful contributions, all of which challenge dominant approaches in the social and natural sciences, and in public health and epidemiology including those that focus on diseases or people in isolation rather than on relations between them.

However, this commonality disguises important points of difference. As will become clear, the authors included in this volume have different views about what it means to study the social organisation of microbial life. Rather than putting forward a unified approach, contributors mobilise contrasting variants of social theory, and have correspondingly diverse ideas about the units of conceptualisation and analysis and about the sorts of questions that could and should be tackled. In what follows we move between alternative positions, not by accident, but in order to fuel debate about the place of practice theory within and as part of a wider repertoire of ideas.

Orientations and approaches

For purists, the roots of 'social practice theory' can be traced back to Bourdieu, Heidegger and Wittgenstein, with authors like Giddens, Schatzki and Reckwitz building on these interpretations and developing them in their own ways. There is no one definition of practice theory or of what sets it apart from other traditions, but proponents usually suppose that practices are distributed across time and space, that they are enacted, reproduced and transformed, that they include or transpire within material arrangements and that they combine to form complexes and bundles.

Not everyone who talks about practices subscribes to these commitments. For some authors, invoking practices rather than individual behaviour underlines the 'social' and shared aspect of what people do. From this perspective, the language of practice helps make sense of when, where and how humans and more-than-humans inter- or intra-act. For those who start from this position, the primary focus is on people and/or more-than-humans, not on the practices they enact or carry. In borrowing concepts from actor network theory and in going along with Latour's (1992) insistence that human and more-than-human actors should be analysed 'symmetrically', contributors including Cusworth et al. and Brown et al. provide new insights into the repair work of contemporary agriculture (seeking to redress the effects of previous strategies), and into the part that architectures and infrastructures play in channelling human and microbial interaction. For these authors, and for others like them, the added value is to treat exchanges between actors (people, infrastructures, microbes) as effects of social practices like tourism or agriculture.

These are important insights, but some contributors go further, arguing that practice theories call for a radical reconceptualisation of how human-microbial relations are established and how they change. This is consistent with the conclusion that practices – distributed across space and time – constitute *the* central topic of investigation and analysis (Giddens, 1984) and with a parallel interest in how 'materials', including more-than-humans, are entangled in the lives of social practices in the arrangements 'amidst which' practices transpire (Schatzki, 2010). Amongst other things, advocates of this approach underline the generative nature of relations between (provisional) entities, arguing that what counts as an 'actor' or a body is itself a product of interactions that are constantly in flux. From this perspective de-centering the human subject is a first step, but the next and in many ways more important challenge is to conceptualise practices and processes that dissolve the 'edges' of discrete entities, whether human or not (see Blue, Chapter 8).

The examples that are discussed in this book – from responses to the body in neonatal care through to encounters with mosquito-borne disease in different locations and from approaches to 'nature' and agriculture to the history of contaminated water – illustrate contrasting ways of thinking about encounters and flows. As such, the collection includes chapters that work with different interpretations of what it means to write about social practices. In a nutshell, some authors refer to practices in order to understand how humans and more-than-humans inter- or intra-act. Meanwhile, others focus on the lives of practices as such, writing about how practices are reproduced and transformed and how they converge and change over time. In the final chapter we return to this issue and to the still-open question of whether contributors undermine or augment existing theoretical approaches.

More straightforwardly, most if not all contributors suppose that microscopic 'materials' could and should figure in social theories of health. In taking up this suggestion, authors consider four themes: contagion, materiality, bodies and concepts of disease, doing so on the grounds that all are important for contemporary forms of epidemiology and public health. Since the four parts of the book are framed by short introductions, each foregrounding areas of overlap and each identifying differences of method and conceptual orientation, the following paragraphs give a very brief account of what the book includes and how it is organised.

Contagion, materiality, bodies, health

In the first part of the book, Shove (Chapter 2) and Broome (Chapter 3) challenge conventional explanations of contagion and resist the temptation to identify causal agents responsible for the spread of disease. Whereas Shove considers the changing complexes of practice of which 'disease situations' (Hinchliffe et al. 2017) are made, Broome describes the circumstances in which people and mosquitos meet, and the practices (for instance of tourism and leisure) on which these meetings depend. In essence, both these authors conclude that it is impossible to understand pathways of infection without also understanding the social practices on which those pathways depend, but they do so for different reasons and in different ways.

The contributions included in the second part of the book also refuse to separate the microbial and the social. Cusworth et al. (Chapter 5), Jauho (Chapter 6) and Brown et al. (Chapter 7) work with different cases and examples – ranging from agriculture to architecture, and encompassing instances of exposure, immunity and disease – doing so in terms that reveal some of the ways in which material and human relations shape and co-constitute each other. Amongst much else, these chapters underline Maller's (Chapter 4) account of the extent to which microbes, some 'good', some 'bad', are implicated in the challenges that humans face today.

The third part of the book has to do with the porosity of the body, and with what that means for the configuration of margins and boundaries, and for the status of people in social theory. Concepts of human exceptionalism depend on the idea that human bodies are neatly demarcated, but what if they are conceived of as crossing points of multiple practices, or as sites of intermingling and flow? In responding to these suggestions, Cohn (Chapter 9) writes about how the boundaries of the body are reproduced and enacted and about how these processes mirror the histories and mixtures of professionals involved (in hospital care). In his contribution, Blue argues that human bodies, along with the microbes that inhabit them (that threaten them or that keep them alive) simultaneously figure as traces and carriers of practice. As Blue (Chapter 8) explains, these conclusions force us to think again about the part that human and more-than-human practitioners play within practice theory and beyond.

The pair of chapters that make up the fourth section deal with discourses and ideas about the causes and characteristics of health and disease at the so-called 'population level'. The first of these two contributions, by Meloni (Chapter 10), provides a history of humoralism, and of contemporary concepts of balance associated with that tradition. The next, by Kelly and Shove (Chapter 11), describes the pervasive power of fundamentally individualistic concepts of contagion, and their impact on the UK government's response to COVID-19. Both authors insist on the usually invisible role of knowledge, broadly defined, and on its performative effect on human and more-than-human actors alike.

In conclusion (Chapter 12), this book captures the novelty and adventure of a field in flux. While most, if not all contributors take issue with received wisdom, and with established ideas about bodies, health and disease, this collection reveals contrasting and sometimes contradictory interpretations of how microbes and societies interact, and of what practice theories have to offer. Readers in search of clear-cut prescriptions for action and intervention may be disappointed, but the tensions we describe are unlikely to disappear any time soon. Rather than striving for some kind of synthesis, this collection is designed to make readers to pause, and to think about what deceptively simple conclusions about the co-constitution of the social and the biological really mean for policy and for research in different disciplines.

References

Barad, K. (2003). 'Posthumanist Performativity: Toward an Understanding of How Matter Comes to Matter', *Signs: Journal of Women in Culture and Society,* 28(3): 801–831.

Barad, K. (2007). *Meeting the universe halfway: quantum physics and the entanglement of matter and meaning.* London: Duke University Press.

Brives, C., Rest, M. and Sariola, S. (eds.) (2021). *With Microbes.* Mattering Press. https://doi.org/10.28938/9781912729180.

Cañada, J. A., Sariola, S. and Butcher, A. (2022). 'In critique of anthropocentrism: a more-than-human ethical framework for antimicrobial resistance', *Medical Humanities,* medhum–2021–012309. https://doi.org/10.1136/medhum-2021-012309.

Giddens, A. (1984). *The Constitution of Society: Outline of the theory of structuration.* Cambridge: Polity Press.

Haraway, D. J. (2008). *When species meet.* Minneapolis: University of Minnesota Press.

Hinchliffe, S., Bingham, N., Allen, J. and Carter, S. (2017). *Pathological* Lives: *Disease, space and biopolitics.* Chichester: England, Wiley.

Latour, B. (1992). 'Where are the missing masses? The sociology of a few mundane artefacts' in Bijker, W. and Law, J. (eds.) *Shaping Technology/Building Society: Studies in Sociotechnical Change.* Cambridge, Mass.: MIT Press: 225–258.

Schatzki, T. (2010). 'Materiality and Social Life', *Nature and Culture,* 5(2): 123–149. https://doi.org/10.3167/nc.2010.050202.

PART I
Framing concepts of contagion

Elizabeth Shove, Cecily Maller and Simon Cohn

The next two chapters are about how diseases travel and where they go. Issues of distribution and spread are not new: epidemiologists, modellers and experts in public health have focused on just this topic and have done so with the help of more and less sophisticated forms of social and spatial mapping and of modelling, including methods of representing complex interactions between habitats, exposures and the reproduction of viruses, bacteria and infectious diseases. Although diverse, these strategies have some features in common, one of which is a tendency to focus on measurable variables including aspects of the 'host' (the person), the infective agent (for example, the mosquito) or the habitats and environments they share.

By contrast, the contributions in this section work with different units of analysis and conceptualisation, arguing that social practices, not individuals, not environments and not social structures constitute what Schatzki (2002) describes as the 'site' of the social. It is this that leads Broome to study the practices that bring people, mosquitos and mosquito-borne diseases together, and this that leads him to describe the overlapping multi-species geographies of encounter and exposure. In Chapter 3, Broome writes about individuals' past experience, matters of timing (when people are around, when mosquitos bite) and the details of how people and insects converge in a park in central Barcelona. In essence, his aim is to develop methods of analysing the social practices on which movements of people, mosquitos and diseases depend, and of studying the intersection of necessarily local conditions (like those that occur in the park), and more extensive trends, in this case, in tourism and leisure.

Broome's focus on practices is novel and generative in that it takes account of factors that are not usually included in epidemiological models, but that

DOI: 10.4324/9781003685210-2

could be. Chapter 2, by Shove shares some of these ideas, also supposing that practices constitute the site of the social. Although this is a common starting point, the two chapters develop in different directions.

In detail, Shove provides a practice-theoretically inspired account of how, where and when situations of encounter and exposure arise. This argues for a more historical approach and for an analysis that emphasises the *ongoing* intermingling of human and non-human life. As described, this is important in that histories of knowledge, including knowledge of disease and its avoidance, are woven into the situations and settings in which people and pathogens meet. In working through these ideas, Shove sets the scene for the chapters that come next, laying the ground for a more comprehensive analysis of flow through and across conventional boundaries, including those that define human and non-human bodies (see Blue, Chapter 8).

Empirically, Shove's strategy is to consider the spread of water-borne disease – cholera in particular – in London from the 1840s to the present day. As she explains, theories about the causes of ill health and its distribution intersect with epidemiological methods and assumptions, and with parallel histories of water, infrastructure and bacteria. Since these understandings are always on the move, the challenge is to show how processes of biosocial becoming create 'disease situations' that are uneven and unequally distributed.

It is tempting to think of trends in public health and in understandings of contagion as expressions and outcomes of external forces including those of capitalism, colonialism or whatever. But for practice theorists such as Shove, Schatzki or Blue, concepts like these do not account for the distribution of infection or the directions in which bodies, viruses and bacteria intermingle. Instead, the claim that disease situations are endogenous and situated outcomes of open-ended processes of reproduction, intersection and amplification goes hand in hand with the further conclusion that what looks like the spread of disease is better understood as the multi-sited enactment of similar configurations of practice.

In some respects, the contributions by Broome and Shove are complementary: both view patterns of exposure as effects of practice and, to varying degrees, both deal with change over time. However, they do not approach this topic in the same way. Broome's method is to describe the geographies of mosquito-human encounter at one moment and in one location. By contrast, Shove focuses on the historical co-evolution of disease situations. These are not incommensurable positions, but they represent one of several moments in the book in which contributors invoke 'stronger' and 'looser' interpretations of practice theory.

These differences aside, the chapters included in the first part of the book challenge and reveal some of the assumptions on which dominant methods of analysis – in epidemiology, in public health – depend. They do so by questioning taken-for-granted variables (some social, some environmental) and upending the terms in which contagion is usually understood. To be clear, this is not just a matter of paying attention to social 'context'. Instead, the stronger argument is that contagion is an effect of the ongoing intermingling of the biosocial, and that this is integral to the long-term dynamics of social practice.

2

CONCEPTUALISING CONTAGION

Disease situations and the histories and geographies of practice

Elizabeth Shove

Introduction

Contagious diseases like the plague, malaria, tuberculosis, cholera and COVID-19 are responsible for death and ill-health on a spectacular scale and it is important to understand how they spread. There are different accounts of transmission, but whether air-borne, water-borne, passed from person to person or carried by insects, it is widely agreed that the geographical distribution of pathogens and their effect on human bodies relates to the social organisation of daily life. This is not a controversial claim, but as one might expect, alternative methods of conceptualising the social and the material generate correspondingly varied interpretations of what contagion involves and how it might be studied and explained.[1]

Having briefly reviewed positions adopted by epidemiologists and by sociologists of science, actor network theorists and those who study more-than-human relations, I suggest that Hinchliffe's ideas about pathogenic landscapes and disease situations (Hinchliffe et al., 2017) open the way for a more subtle account of the spatial distribution of microscopic matter and of human and non-human intra-action. I illustrate this potential with reference to a discussion of water infrastructures and water-borne disease in London from the 1850s to the present. As I go on to show, social theories of practice, as developed by authors such as Schatzki (2002), Reckwitz (2002), Shove, Blue and Kelly (2024), help make sense of how disease situations arise and of the complexes of social, material and microbial arrangements on which contagion depends. As represented here, practice theories provide a means of bridging between those who focus on the social construction of knowledge, the materiality of the social world and the implications of both

DOI: 10.4324/9781003685210-3

for the histories and geographies of contagious disease. More than that, they underpin what might become a new style of epidemiology, treating social practices, not people and not microbes, as the site of the biosocial (Ingold, 2013) and contagion as an outcome of doings and sayings, distributed across space and time.

The social and the microbial: Concepts of contagion

Although this is where the chapter leads, my first step is to take stock of some of the ways in which social and microbial worlds have been understood and what these interpretations mean for ideas about infectious diseases and how they spread.

It makes sense to start with a few words about epidemiology, a discipline that is centrally concerned with questions about where and how people and pathogens meet. Epidemiology is a huge and complicated field, but in modelling relations between hosts, agents and environments, epidemiologists are, for the most part, interested in isolating the causes of disease and in identifying subsets of the population that are more or less at risk. The list of variables is different but whether the problem is that of understanding the spread of cholera in London in the 1840s, or of COVID-19 in the 2020s, the basic approach is similar. In both cases, and in many others besides, there is a shared tendency to boil the social world down to a set of conditions associated with unequal patterns of exposure to identifiable bacteriological or viral threats. In reflecting on this tendency, Kelly and Russo recognise that 'It is not uncommon to find the social being articulated in medical investigations, but it is seldom foregrounded and usually plays a role as context, or in how epidemiology variables like age, gender, occupation are used' (Kelly and Russo, 2021: 116). The specification of the microbial world is similarly bounded, focusing on identifiable pathogens, as these are known and understood at any one moment in time.

In essence, conventional epidemiological methods treat the social, the material and the biological as separate and identifiable factors, not as aspects of a more fluid, constantly evolving complex. As a result, they tend to overlook the longer-term histories of microbial and human interaction and the ideas and paradigms on which these arrangements depend. Patterns of infection are consequently conceptualised as outcomes of the spatial conjunction of hosts, agents and environments, the distribution of which is attributed to measurable factors including demographic or 'social' variables.

By contrast, sociologists of scientific knowledge take a much broader view of what counts as social, arguing that theories about natural, biological, physical and chemical processes are framed by beliefs, methods and understandings that are related to institutions, funding regimes, careers and priorities (Kuhn, 1970). From this point of view, ideas about bacteria, viruses and biological processes are always of their time. To give a couple of examples, studies that investigate the details of laboratory life (Latour and Woolgar, 1986), or that show how distinctions between things of nature (for example cells) and man-made technologies are constituted and changed, show how microbiological research agendas are shaped by political and commercial concerns (Landecker, 2006).

The conclusion that histories of scientific enquiry are entangled in social relations and that these matter for the development and circulation of concepts and methods does not mean that the 'material' world is somehow missing. In *The Pasteurisation of France* (1993), Latour argues that microscopic entities represent emerging partners in the making of germ theory and in the enactment of germ-inspired ways of life. In effect, Latour positions Pasteur and Pasteurians as spokespersons for non-human actors, and for populations of bacteria. As he explains, representing microscopic 'animals' and their 'aims', and responding to them, depends on a network of convinced scientists, controversies, institutional arrangements and material alliances.

Latour does not say much about how theories and diseases spread, but he argues that once belief in the existence of invisible 'creatures' took hold, it became clear that society was 'not made up just of men' ... and that ... 'everywhere microbes intervene and act' (Latour, 1993: 35). In characterising these interactions, Latour describes connections between separate and distinct entities: that is between germs, people and their understandings of the microbial world.

Other lines of enquiry take the social organisation of knowledge for granted, putting the history of ideas in the background and focusing instead on how human and more-than-human entities shape each other now and in the recent past. Biologists, anthropologists, geographers and feminist researchers who write about diet and digestion (Paxson, 2023), fermentation (special issue of *Current Anthropology* (Rutherford, 2021), or composting (Abrahamsson and Bertoni, 2014) are, for instance, interested in the effects that industrialisation, capitalism or colonialism have on human and non-human interactions. Landecker's pathbreaking study of the rise of antimicrobial resistance is a good example. In an article entitled 'Antibiotic Resistance and the Biology of History', Landecker (2016) argues that resistance is an outcome of an ongoing cycle in which intensive farming comes to depend on antibiotics, and in which bacteria adapt to widespread and highly selective attempts to kill them. Tracy's (2021) account of cows as machines for making milk takes much the same approach, also invoking generic theories of economic power and also supposing that non-human actants (such as bacteria and viruses) are capable of kicking back and influencing the course of human history.

Paxson and Helmreich conclude that studies of this kind have the double effect of showing how communities of microscopic organisms are 'mediated by social rules but also by (micro)biopolitics, capitalism, and technoscience'

(Paxson, 2023: 7) and of revealing the 'cultural, social, political, and scientific practices that microbes tend to reformat and reshuffle... in unexpected ways' (Paxson and Helmreich, 2014: 167). This is consistent with what actor network theorists describe as a 'symmetrical' method, this being one that takes the material, and in this case, the non- or more-than-human, on a par with social – that is human – life. In addition, and as indicated above, some authors claim that social-microbial interactions are defined by political and economic forces and that these are crucial for where and how infections spread. Whether they share this view or not, proponents of more-than-human studies are broadly agreed that biological and social processes shape each other, and that patterns and pathways of contagion mirror these interactions.

As these various interpretations suggest, ideas about the social and the microbial are crucial for how contagion is understood, and for how diseases are thought to spread. More specifically, symmetrical accounts of how human and more-than-human relations constitute each other differ from epidemiological traditions in which 'social factors' are treated as background features that affect the incidence of disease, but that are not affected by it.

There are, of course, other possible positions, but before moving on it is useful to pause for a moment and take stock of the strategies outlined above. To recap, I began by noticing that conventional epidemiological methods treat contagion and the geographical spread of infection as an outcome of the socioeconomic characteristics of different sectors of the population, the properties of different sorts of infective 'agents' and the environments they inhabit. In focusing on factors and variables, proponents of these traditions tend to overlook the histories of social and microbial interaction and take little or no account of changing paradigms.

By contrast, authors who study the social organisation of scientific knowledge, including that which is developed and enacted by people in their role as spokespersons for microscopic entities, suppose that social arrangements matter for how microbiological knowledge is produced. More than that, they contend that this is of practical significance because ideas (for example, about humours, germs and so forth) are crucial for the lives of bacteria and viruses, for related infrastructures and practices, for when, where and how people and pathogens encounter each other, and for how contagious diseases spread.

These insights are relevant for research that focuses, symmetrically, on how human and more-than-human beings are embedded in social and material worlds that are jointly shaped by external forces including those of capitalism, colonialism and industrialisation. From this perspective, understanding contagion is a matter of understanding how the geographies of infection relate to the uneven political and economic geographies of risk and exposure.

The underlying rationale and the purpose and direction of enquiry differ, but the approaches sketched above are alike in identifying connections between what are thought to be bounded entities (people, bacteria), even when the substance of those categories changes, and even when entities are thought to interact and shape each other. This is not the only path to follow and, as outlined below, social theories of practice provide another way of thinking about the microbial and the social and thus about the spread of infectious disease.

There are many varieties of practice theory and prominent authors including Bourdieu, Giddens, Schatzki and Reckwitz, disagree on a number of counts. However, all take social practices to be the basic units of conceptualisation and analysis. For these writers, practice *theory* involves much more than an interest in what people do. Many (but not all) practice theorists subscribe to a series of connected propositions: that practices exist across space and time, 'that practices consist in organised sets of actions, that practices link to form wider complexes and constellations' (Hui et al., 2017: 2), that this nexus represents the 'basic domain of study of the social sciences' (Giddens, 1984: 2) and that practices are what there is to social life, meaning there are no higher levels of explanation.

These commitments set practice theorists apart from those who focus on individuals' beliefs and choices, or who suppose that social life is governed by external political or economic forces, or by contextual or environmental factors. A further feature, and one that is especially important in the present context, is that material elements (Shove et al., 2012) and/or material arrangements (Schatzki, 2010) are taken to be integral to the lives of practices. This implies that practices are not just the site of the social (Schatzki, 2002), as a distinct sphere of human activity, but that they are also the site of what Ingold describes as the biosocial (Ingold, 2013). As Ingold insists, the biosocial is not some hybrid term in which the social and the biological represent separate worlds that interact. Instead, his much stronger conclusion is that what are usually treated as distinct realms are thoroughly intermingled. This is a critical insight, and one that is important for social theory and for theories of practice in particular.

It is so in that it reminds us that the domain of the material includes microscopic particles of organic and inorganic matter, the definition and status of which are interwoven discursively and in practice. Putting these pieces together, and following Ingold's lead, it makes sense to conclude that the distribution and history of bacteria, viruses and other pathogens are rooted in the plenum of practice. Although practice theorists have yet to say much about the microscopic world or about contagion and disease, many would agree that humans, more-than-humans and micromaterials of all kinds carry and also transform complexes of practice *and* the ideas and understandings associated with them. This is in keeping with the claim that discursive and material arrangements combine to form configurations that are crucial for the histories and geographies of infection.

In order to bring these rather abstract suggestions to life, the next part of the chapter shows what different theories and approaches mean for ideas about correlation, causation and the conditions in which infection occurs.

Causes, complexes and disease situations

In what follows, I take John Snow's famous study of cholera as a point of departure and as a point of reference for an increasingly complicated discussion of disease situations and of the practices on which these situations depend.

As is widely known, Snow plotted instances of the disease in the Soho area of London in 1854 and correlated these with the consumption of water drawn from the Broad Street pump. Removing the handle of the pump coincided with a decline in the outbreak, lending weight to Snow's theory that cholera was water-borne and not transmitted through the air, as was previously thought.

Some claim that Snow's study laid the foundations for contemporary epidemiology but as others point out, similar statistical methods were already in use, including techniques developed by William Farr. There is also much debate about the rigour of Snow's research, and especially about the data he used and his failure to record population density or the trajectory of the disease over time (Koch, 2014). Setting these critiques aside, Snow's study is revealing in that it focuses on the (then) current incidence of cholera, and on a limited list of variables, linked to ideas about water and its role as a means of transmission. On this point, it is important to note that Snow asked victims about sources of water supply, but not about the air they breathed, who they met or what they wore. In this respect, and in others, his investigation was evidently framed by, and evidently designed to counter, miasmatic theories of air-borne transmission. As these few comments suggest, Snow's research represents a moment in a long-running history of ideas and in related methods of bounding and studying the spread of disease (Amsterdamska, 2005).

There are parallels between germ theory and Snow's version of epidemiology in that both suppose that there are identifiable causal agents, and that risks of exposure and contagion can be isolated and quantified. Snow's study, and the styles of epidemiology that it has inspired, move between observed correlations and the identification of critical connections – in Snow's case, mapping cases of cholera and linking them to source of water supply narrowed the list of possible causes. However, investigations like these do not show how concepts like those of cleanliness and dirt evolved, how water was in any case piped to the Broad Street pump or what it was used for in the home. In so far as they figure at all, these features form part of the background, or environment in which contagion occurs.

As experts in public health are keen to point out, noticing correlations is not the same as identifying causal relations. Equally, specifying the mechanisms involved, and in this case, isolating the bacteria responsible for cholera, does not of itself explain patterns and pathways of contagion. In addition, and in some ways more important, none of these approaches reveal the dynamics of the situation. As we now know, outbreaks of cholera in Broad Street and elsewhere formed part of an ongoing and unfolding process of biosocial change in which some people died of cholera, some didn't catch it at all, and some did but then survived. Through all of this, Vibrio cholerae continued to evolve.

Hamlin (2009), who is an historian, and geographers like Hinchliffe et al. (2017), take up this theme, arguing that patterns of immunity, resistance and response – human and microbial – are outcomes of integrated and dynamic processes and of 'pathogenic landscapes' shaped by the multiple conditions and circumstances in which diverse social groups and populations of bacteria and viruses intermingle. Rather than trying to pin down causal factors, these authors conclude that contagion 'is the outcome of a continuous interplay between animals, microbes, people and materials that intraact as they circulate, producing a shifting and a more or less pathogenic landscape' (Hinchliffe et al., 2017: 112). By implication, it is the interplay that counts, not the relation between bounded variables, as if these were separate, or separable from the settings in which they occur. In addition, and as Hinchliffe et al. (2017) and Hamlin (2009) insist, disease biographies are inherently fluid. By implication, cholera arises within and because of an extensive complex of human and more-than-human arrangements *all* of which are important for when, where and how the disease spreads and for what it becomes.

To go back to the Broad Street pump, in the 1850s piped water was drawn from the river Thames just a mile or so away. But as historians and geographers point out, trends in water consumption, and ideas about contagion extend beyond the city itself. For example, Massey (2005) and Hinchliffe (2024) argue that any one location is made by the intersection of overlapping practices, past and present. When seen in these terms, outbreaks of cholera in London's Soho, were not 'just' effects of biological infection or of exclusively local encounters: they were outcomes of a multitude of situated co-requisites, vulnerabilities and exposures and of ideas and material relations, some of which were reproduced in other places as well.

Assuming the Broad Street pump was a source of contaminated water and of cholera, it was so because of how it fitted into a much wider infrastructure of consumption and provision. From this perspective, the very existence of the pump, the arrangements that made it possible, the underground pipes leading to it, the buckets and pails in which water was carried away, the economics of supply and the practicalities of demand (how often was the pump visited, and by whom) were necessary but invisible parts of the 'disease situation' that pertained at the time (Hinchliffe et al., 2017).

Hinchliffe et al. elaborate on this conclusion, suggesting that a disease situation is

> at once grounded somewhere but also dispersed or distributed through the many interactions that make it [disease] possible and which it can also affect. For us, situations are meeting places, where numerous actors, bodies, species, pressures, flows, issues, decisions and so on are organised or brought together, or held apart or worked upon. They are heterogeneous (formed from their differences and relations), and dependent for their identity not only on what is meeting up but also how those meetings are configured.
>
> *(Hinchliffe et al., 2017: 33)*

Capturing these interactions and their impact on the geography of contagion arguably depends on an account of microorganisms, not as discrete causal factors but as momentary traces of practices as they extend and change.

This is obvious if we think about how water supplies in Soho have evolved. The area that Snow described is now served by networks of water treatment and provision, and by sewerage systems defined and governed by diverse patterns of investment, regulation and ownership. In 2006, Thames Water, which is currently responsible for supplying Soho, became part of the Kemble Water Group, financed by a consortium of institutional shareholders the largest of which is a Canadian pension fund. Alongside this mesh of commercial interests, levels of service provision and costs are regulated by the Water Services Regulation Authority (Ofwat), established in 1989. Other changes, including the expectation that homes will be equipped with taps and indoor plumbing, and that water will be safe to drink, matter for the scale of demand, for methods of water treatment and for related forms of microbial encounter (Tomory, 2017).

Contemporary systems of provision and methods of treating and chlorinating water mean that in central London, cholera is, for now, a thing of the past. This is so despite the fact that some parts of the water infrastructure date back to the Victorian period and before, that other parts, such as the new 'super sewer', also known as London's Tideway Tunnel, are much more recent and that per capita consumption has increased substantially since the 1850s. In London, as in other locations, histories of technology and of ownership and governance do not just stop and there is no reason to suppose that future systems of provision will be the same as those of today, or that patterns of cost and responsibility will remain unchanged. Equally, there is no blank slate, meaning that water-related disease situations emerge from, and relate to material, institutional and ideological complexes and to the lives of the many practices involved.

This far I have focused on water, and on systems of provision and patterns of demand and I have done so in order to distinguish between Snow's epidemiological method, and Hinchliffe's analysis of disease situations. As described above, Snow sought to isolate the causes of cholera by plotting the social and spatial distribution of the disease. This allowed him to trace the source of infection back to the Broad Street pump, but it revealed little, if anything, about the history of water provision and consumption or about the multiple geographies on which outbreaks of cholera depend. In essence, Snow's method describes provisionally stable environments in which identifiable hosts and agents meet. There are, of course, contemporary forms of epidemiological modelling that make use of complexity theory and that seek to describe a mass of interdependent relations, but at the end of the day they also revolve around the analysis of discrete and bounded entities. By contrast, Hinchliffe is interested in the constitution and distribution of situations that are entangled, geographically diverse, and historically variable.

In the next and final part of the chapter, I suggest that Hinchliffe's account of pathogenic landscapes is compatible with aspects of science studies, actor network theory, and contemporary forms of feminism and anthropology, and that social theories of practice provide a means of drawing these contributions together. This is an important exercise in that it depends on an account of social-microbial intermingling that confounds the purifying work of abstracting variables and causal factors, and that lays the ground for a more situational and also more dynamic version of epidemiology, not as we know it today but as it might become.

Integrating ideas

I began by outlining different methods of conceptualising social and microbial life and of understanding how infectious diseases spread. This included a brief review of conventional epidemiological methods compared with those that foreground the production of scientific knowledge, or that insist on the symmetrical treatment of human and more-than-human life, mediated by systems like those of capitalism, colonialism or industrialisation.

In bringing the chapter to a close I expand on the further suggestion that the spread, or more accurately, the multi-sited reproduction of disease situations is an outcome of how practices are distributed and how they combine now, and in the past. This is not a unique or especially novel contribution. In his impressive account of the 'biography' of cholera, Hamlin takes a similar approach, describing the changing characteristics of *Vibrio cholerae* and the interventions and strategies associated with its ongoing career (Hamlin,

2009). Rather than supposing that cholera is a stable entity that moves from one place to another (as Snow does and as epidemiologists generally do), Hamlin's biographical method is consistent with the claim that patterns of contagion depend on multiple practices and on how these combine and change.

Although Hamlin does not make the link in quite these terms, his work supports the conclusion that widespread trends – for instance in ideas about infection and the geographical distribution of harmful bacteria – are effects of overlapping histories and arrangements, including relations between pumps, watercourses, patterns of urban planning, investment and demand. This is in keeping with the view that the distribution and co-evolution of human and more-than-human life depends on an unbroken sequence in which past complexes of microscopic materials, diseases and practices are relevant for those of the present and in which current configurations matter for the future. Analytically this turns the spotlight back on to questions about how practices connect, spatially and over time (Shove, 2023).

These are not new concerns. For example, Schatzki (2016a) considers the emergence of widespread and in that sense 'large' social phenomena, identifying forms of hybridisation and accumulation and their consequences for the geographical distribution of practices including those that constitute the habitats in which organisms and microbes coexist and that define the sites in which contagion occurs. For Schatzki, and for others, practices are always 'local' in that they are instantiated and enacted in specific settings. Technically, this means that complexes of practice do not literally spread – instead, they are recurrently and similarly enacted in multiple locations. It is on this basis that Hinchliffe et al. conclude that a disease situation is 'a trans-species, multi-sited matter where practices and orderings are more-than-human affairs and pathogenicity is produced from an array of seemingly complex interrelations' (Hinchliffe et al., 2017: 105). As these authors go on to explain,

> Pathogens, when seen in this light, do not simply spread out from a mappable location or source, and nor do they merely diffuse across space. They intraact (to reuse Barad's term (Barad, 2007)) to the extent that they not only mutate as they move, they also drift and shift through all manner of transfections, transductions and transformations.
>
> *(Hinchliffe et al., 2017: 106)*

To be clear, the point is not just that epidemics and outbreaks need to be understood as 'multiple, overlapping phenomena with many meanings' (Herring and Swedlund, 2010: 24). That is so, but the further suggestion is that multi-species encounters and adaptations depend on habitats defined and constituted by constantly evolving packages of practice (Green, 2015).

In other words, contagion happens within and as part of a differentiated and bumpy landscape of possibility, shaped by the unequally distributed residues and traces of biosocial configurations. Since packages of practice are simultaneously localised and geographically overlapping, they constitute disease situations some of which are similar, or similar enough to sustain the notion of spread, and to support the view that infections 'travel' from one location to the next.

The distinction between strategies that focus on multiple sites of enactment, on the one hand, or on generic mechanisms of contagion, on the other, is of more than academic concern. As we know, competing theories of contagion matter for what happens next, and for the characteristics and qualities of public and private efforts to limit exposure and the risk of disease. As already mentioned, there is a tendency to attribute the changing contours of contagion (and/or immunity and resistance) to political and economic systems associated with capitalism, colonialism etc. and to suppose that these systems have an existence of their own. Anderson is, for instance, of the view that it is possible to identify 'underlying structures and dynamic modifications in our societies and environments that promote or retard the emergence and spread of infectious disease' (Anderson, 2021: 178).

'Strong' practice theorists, including Schatzki and Shove adopt what is known as a flat ontology, meaning that they do not accept that there are higher levels of explanation. In Schatzki's words, 'Practice ontologies are flat because (1) they treat practices as the central element in the constitution of social phenomena; and (2) practices are laid out on one level' (Schatzki, 2016b: 31). Accordingly, 'One mark of the flatness of these ontologies is that they analyse social phenomena as arrays of the components of fields, systems, bundles/complexes, or plenum and as lacking any substantive or distinct existence beyond this' (Schatzki, 2016b: 31). This is relevant in that those who subscribe to a flat ontology resist the conclusion that patterns of contagion are indicative of some external force. It is obviously possible to describe pathogenic landscapes and aspects of disease situations that are widely shared, but for practice theorists, the point is that these are emergent and contingent patterns, and not expressions of something else. There is, of course, some direction to the ways in which practices unfold but as Schatzki explains, practices and complexes of them have histories and geographies of their own, and it is these that matter for how biosocial phenomena develop and change, and for how infections spread.

Bringing these ideas together, a practice theoretically compatible account of contagion (or multi-sited enactment) would a) take heed of the dynamic features of disease situations and pathogenic landscapes b) focus on the discourses, material arrangements and practices of which these situations are made; and c) show how distributions and accumulations of materials (whether human or more-than-human) affect the lives of practices and where they occur. In short, such an account would revolve around a multi-sited analysis of how practices extend, converge and change.

Neighbouring fields, including actor network theory, the sociology of scientific knowledge, feminism and anthropology and various styles of political, economic and biological theory address aspects of this agenda. As outlined above, they take note of changing histories of ideas, they acknowledge the importance of symmetrical accounts of human and microbial interaction, and they foreground what are taken to be widespread features of contemporary society, including those of intensive agriculture, standardised diets and so forth. These are useful contributions but taking practices – not microbes, not people, not 'actor networks' and not political and economic systems – as the central topic of conceptualisation and enquiry changes the questions that are asked and the terms in which they are addressed. It does so in that the presence or absence of contagious disease is viewed as an outcome of the social organisation not only of knowledge, or of material-human interaction, but of the historical and geographical trajectories of entire complexes of practice.

In theory these ideas might inspire new ways of thinking about the distribution of risk and contagion, and about conjunctions of practices, and the materials (including micromaterials) and discourses on which these depend. Whether they do so or not remains to be seen, but the potential is there.

By contrast, and for the time being, public health interventions tend to focus on specific threats and on means of avoiding them or limiting their impact (see Kelly and Shove, Chapter 11). As with Snow's study of cholera, these strategies have the necessary and parallel effect of obscuring crucial features of the historically and geographically variable situations in which people and microbes evolve together. To some extent, this kind of bounding is needed in order to figure out what constitutes a disease situation (as opposed to a 'situation' of some other kind) and to identify the sorts of interactions on which specifically *pathogenic* landscapes depend. However, it is vital to remember that enquiries of this kind proceed by leaving out co-requisites, co-existing conditions, and most important of all, the dynamics of social practice on which biosocial relations depend.

One response is to fold these considerations back in, and to describe disease biographies as Hamlin does, or to map out the features of pathogenic landscapes, as Hinchliffe does, and to think about how these develop together. Proponents of 'historical epidemiology' come close in aiming to show how 'interventions have transformed patterns of disease and influenced disease transmission' (Webb, 2015: 322). As Webb describes, the further ambition is to bring the historical and spatial features of human-pathogen relations into view.

Another response is to argue that the challenge is not simply one of integrating multiple processes (ecological, social, economic and political) in order to provide a more holistic account of microbial life. Instead (and following Ingold, 2013) a comprehensively biosocial analysis depends on overcoming ready-made distinctions between the biological and the social. This calls for methods not (or not only) of bounding, narrowing and purification but of describing how complexes of practices and social-microbial interminglings arise, extend and change. By implication, interventions – including that of removing the handle of the Broad Street pump – are interventions in a stream of ongoing relations and configurations, combinations of which constitute 'local' and also 'global' processes of becoming on which patterns of contagion depend. What is missing, but what theories of practice offer, is a means of understanding these provisional and situated aspects of contagion.

Finally, and more by way of a postscript than a definitive ending, it is as well to remember that social theories – including those discussed above – are integrated into the worlds they describe. Methods and concepts are never innocent and all forms of knowing are political in that they rely on some but not other commitments and conventions. This is important in that ideas are performative, meaning that they are inscribed in policies and practices, including those of farming, cleaning, treating water and providing advice about public health.

By way of example, contemporary methods of modelling the spread of infectious disease are frequently founded on the belief that health phenomena are

> linked to behaviors and interactions: mainly relationships between individuals (contacts, spatial proximity relationships, behavioral relationships) or relationships between individuals and their environment (natural, social, economic, etc.).
>
> *(Souris, 2019: 1)*

These assumptions are hard-wired into research and into measures designed to improve or protect public health and as such they have real if unpredictable consequences within and as part of the flux of biosocial becoming.

Other ways of thinking about the social and microbial world would have different consequences, and they would also feed into the dynamic processes of which human and non- or more-than-human lives are made. It is impossible to anticipate the difference that a practice theoretically compatible account of contagion might make, but if this approach were to catch on, and if it was to become part of the lives of people and of bacteria and viruses, it would also become part of the ongoing dynamics that it describes.

Note

1 Technically, contagion refers to transmission that happens between people, with infection being the more generic concept. In what follows, I take a looser approach, using both terms to describe the changing geographies of organisms and pathogenic microbes.

References

Abrahamsson, S. and Bertoni, F. (2014). 'Compost Politics: Experimenting with Togetherness in Vermicomposting', *Environmental humanities*, 4(1): 125–148. https://doi.org/10.1215/22011919-3614962.

Amsterdamska, O. (2005). 'Demarcating Epidemiology', *Science, technology and human values*, 30(1): 17–51. https://doi.org/10.1177/0162243904270719.

Anderson, W. (2021). 'The model crisis, or how to have critical promiscuity in the time of Covid-19', *Social Studies of Science*, 51(2): 167–188. https://doi.org/10.1177/0306312721996053.

Barad, K. (2007). *Meeting the Universe Halfway: Quantum physics and the entanglement of matter and meaning*. London: Duke University Press.

Giddens, A. (1984) *The Constitution of Society: Outline of the Theory of Structuration*, Cambridge: Polity Press.

Green, M. (2015). 'The Black Death and Ebola: On the value of comparison' in Green, M. (ed) *Pandemic Disease in the Medieval World: Rethinking the black death*. Kalamazoo: Arc Medieval Press.

Hamlin, C. (2009). *Cholera: The biography*. Oxford: Oxford University Press.

Herring, D. and Swedlund, A. (2010). 'Plagues and epidemics in anthropological perspective' in Herring, D. and Swedlund, A. (eds.) *Plagues and Epidemics: Infected spaces, past and present*. Oxford: Taylor and Francis Group. 18–36. https://doi.org/10.4324/9781003086376.

Hinchliffe, S. (2024). 'Politics, Space and the More-than-Human Condition' in Franklin, A., (ed) *The Routledge International Handbook of More-than-Human Studies*. London: Routledge. 129–140.

Hinchliffe, S., Bingham, N., Allen, J. and Carter, S. (2017). *Pathological Lives: Disease, space and biopolitics*. Chichester: Wiley.

Hui, A., Schatzki, T. and Shove, E. (eds.) (2017). *The Nexus of Practices: Connections, constellations, practitioners*, London: Routledge. https://doi.org/10.4324/9781315560816.

Ingold, T. (2013). 'Prospect' in Ingold, T. and Pálsson, G. (eds.) *Biosocial Becomings: Integrating social and biological anthropology*. Cambridge: Cambridge University Press. 1–21. https://doi.org/10.1017/CBO9781139198394.

Kelly, M. P. and Russo, F. (2021). 'The epistemic values at the basis of epidemiology and public health'. *Mefisto* 5(1): 105–110. https://doi.org/10.4454/mefisto.5-1.

Koch, T. (2014). 'Commentary: Nobody loves a critic: Edmund A Parkes and John Snow's cholera'. *International Journal of Epidemiology* 42(6): 1553–1559. https://doi.org/10.1093/ije/dyt194.

Kuhn, T. (1970). *The Structure of Scientific Revolutions*. Chicago: University of Chicago Press.

Landecker, H. (2006). *Culturing Life: How cells became technologies*. Cambridge MA: Harvard University Press.

Landecker, H. (2016). 'Antibiotic Resistance and the Biology of History', *Body and Society*, 22: 19–52. https://doi.org/10.1177/1357034X14561341.
Latour, B. (1993). *The Pasteurization of France.* Cambridge MA: Harvard University Press.
Latour, B. and Woolgar, S. (1986). *Laboratory Life: The construction of scientific facts.* Princeton, NJ: Princeton University Press.
Massey, D. (2005). *For Space.* London: Sage.
Paxson, H. (2023). (ed) *Eating Beside Ourselves: Thresholds of foods and bodies.* Durham: Duke University Press. https://doi.org/10.1215/9781478024064.
Paxson, H. and Helmreich, S. (2014). 'The perils and promises of microbial abundance: Novel natures and model ecosystems, from artisanal cheese to alien seas', *Social Studies of Science,* 44(2): 165–193. https://doi.org/10.1177/0306312713505003.
Reckwitz, A. (2002). 'Toward a Theory of Social Practices: A Development in Culturalist Theorizing', *European Journal of Social Theory*, 5(2): 243–263. https://doi.org/10.4324/9781315560816.
Rutherford, D. (2021). 'Cultures of Fermentation: Wenner-Gren Symposium Supplement 24', *Current Anthropology*, 62(S24): S193–S196.
Schatzki, T. (2002). *The Site of the Social: A philosophical account of the constitution of social life and change.* Pennsylvania State University Press: University Park, PA.
Schatzki, T. (2010). 'Materiality and Social Life', *Nature and Culture,* 5(2): 123–149. https://doi.org/10.3167/nc.2010.050202.
Schatzki, T. (2016a). 'Keeping Track of Large Phenomena', *Geographische Zeitschrift,* 104(1): 4–24. http://www.jstor.org/stable/45173996.
Schatzki, T. (2016b). 'Practice theory as a flat ontology' in Spaargaren, G., Weenink, D. and Lamers, M. (eds.) *Practice Theory and Research: Exploring the dynamics of social life.* London: Routledge. 28–43.
Shove, E. (2023). *Connecting Practices: Large topics in society and social theory.* London: Routledge. https://doi.org/10.4324/9781003275107.
Shove, E., Blue, S. and Kelly, M. P. (2024). 'Categorising and cohabiting: practices as the site of biosocial becoming', *Social theory and health,* 22(2): 156–171. https://doi.org/10.1057/s41285-024-00204-7.
Shove, E., Pantzar, M. and Watson, M. (2012). *The Dynamics of Social Practice: Everyday life and how it changes.* London: Sage. https://doi.org/10.4135/9781446250655.
Souris, M. (2019). *Epidemiology and Geography: Principles, Methods and Tools of Spatial Analysis*, Newark: Wiley.
Tomory, L. (2017). *The History of the London Water Industry 1580–1820.* Baltimore: Johns Hopkins University Press.
Tracy, M. (2021). 'Missing Microbes and Other Gendered Microbiopolitics in Bovine Fermentation', *Current Anthropology*, 62(S24): S276–S286. https://doi.org/10.1086/714345.
Webb, J. (2015). 'The historical epidemiology of global disease challenges', *The Lancet*, 385(9965): 322–323. https://doi.org/10.1016/s0140-6736(15)60108-8.

3

PRACTICES, SPACES AND SPECIES

Rethinking human–mosquito interactions and disease transmission

Karl Broome

Introduction

Mosquito-borne diseases (MBDs) represent a significant and growing public health concern, exacerbated by anthropogenic climate change, global mobility and trade (including the circulation of used tires and plants), and processes of urbanisation (Willoughby et al., 2022). Despite global campaigns and substantial investment in public health responses, dominant approaches to mosquito control often prioritise individual behaviour modification through awareness campaigns, or technological solutions such as chemical insecticides, genetic modification, vaccines, and an expanding range of surveillance systems (Biehler et al., 2019). Approaches that seek to incorporate 'social factors' into understanding mosquito habitat formation, exposure and MBD transmission typically draw on concepts such as social-structural determinants or behavioural heterogeneity, generally grounded in aggregated individual-level data. Moreover, data on human 'behaviour' related to MBDs are largely produced through surveys, including Knowledge, Attitude, and Practices (KAP) assessments. While undoubtedly important, these frameworks tend to overlook the complex, relational dynamics of human–mosquito interactions as they are embedded in situated practices, and the role these interactions play in MBD exposure and transmission.

In the field of evolutionary biology, it is usual to focus on changing relations between three key factors: the vector, the pathogen and the host. For example, Powell argues that

> vector-borne diseases represent a three-species interaction problem. The interconnectedness of the three players (vector, pathogen, vertebrate) is

DOI: 10.4324/9781003685210-4

> the outcome of coevolutionary processes acting, in some cases, over long periods of time and, in other cases, very short periods of time.
>
> *(Powell, 2019: 1)*

By contrast, authors who subscribe to more complex and more relational approaches argue that this 'dance of agency' (Pickering, 1995) always involves more than three players. That is to say, MBDs are always more than a three-species interaction problem. This is obvious for authors who are interested in the so-called 'social factors' of exposure and in how these relate to mosquito-borne disease and public health.

As outlined below, it is not usual to frame these issues in terms of practices. In what follows I explore that potential and show what this means for the terms in which exposure and spread are conceptualised and for how interventions are imagined and enacted.

The chapter is structured as follows. First, it provides some background on the tiger mosquito, including its environmental preferences and behavioural repertoires. It then outlines the growing emphasis on social complexity in existing public health and epidemiological approaches. Next, it considers how scholars working within critical social theory and the humanities have reframed disease ecologies and exposure through relational and more-than-human perspectives. The chapter then introduces a selection of concepts drawn from practice theory, before bringing some of these ideas to bear on a study on human-mosquito interaction in Catalonia. The chapter concludes by considering some of the methodological and practical implications of this approach.

Mosquito-borne diseases in an urbanising world

MBDs like dengue, chikungunya, Zika and West Nile virus present considerable global health challenges, particularly in urban settings. The tiger mosquito, *Aedes albopictus*, originally from Southeast Asia and now present on every continent except Antarctica, epitomises this risk. Its urban adaptability, specifically its propensity to breed in small water containers (e.g., plant pots, dumped tires, discarded plastic, styrofoam cups, buckets, irrigation sources), gives it competitive superiority over most other species, and its preference for human hosts contributes to the public health significance of this aggressive daytime biter (Rose et al., 2020).

While the tiger mosquito's flight range is typically limited to 200 metres, human mobility plays an important role in disseminating both mosquitoes and the viruses they carry across various scales, from neighbourhoods to international borders, thereby establishing new contact zones (Beisel and Wergin, 2022). The so-called transmission cycle begins when a female mosquito, requiring a blood meal for egg development, bites an infected human. The ingested pathogen then replicates within the mosquito, eventually migrating to its salivary glands. Subsequent bites can then transmit the virus to new human hosts, completing the cycle.

Not all bites from infected mosquitoes lead to infection, nor do all infected individuals become symptomatic. Several factors are thought to influence why mosquitoes prefer to bite some people more than others, such as having blood type O (Shirai et al., 2004) or the composition of skin bacteria (Michalet et al., 2019). Although *Aedes albopictus* bites during daylight hours, its peak activity at dawn and dusk significantly increases the risk of exposure during the early morning and late afternoon.

The geographical spread of *Aedes albopictus* across Europe has expanded, leading to periodic outbreaks, and raising urgent public health concerns (García-San-Miguel et al., 2024). MBDs, for which the tiger mosquito acts as a vector, not only compromise individual health but can also disrupt daily life, local economies, and vital industries such as tourism (Biehler et al., 2019). Tourism, which is the focus of this chapter, consequently, figures in multiple ways: as a 'carrier' of infection and as a source of urban and environmental change.

On the first point, tourists are known to carry infections from one place to another. While West Nile Virus (WNV) is endemic in Spain, the risk posed by Chikungunya, Zika and Dengue Fever is on the rise. Notably, recent autochthonous dengue cases have been identified among tourists returning from popular European destinations, including the Spanish island of Ibiza (García-San-Miguel et al., 2024). Since 2015, all dengue cases in Spain have been mandatorily reported to the National Epidemiological Surveillance Network (RENAVE), with most infections originating from travellers returning from dengue-endemic regions (Herrero-Martínez et al., 2023: 3).

Another way in which mosquito-borne diseases intersect with tourism practices is through what Gössling (2002) describes as 'leisure-related environmental alterations'. These encompass changes in land cover and land use, the trans-geographical movement of biota, and the spread of diseases.

These are not the only factors involved, but both are important in the examples discussed below.

Social complexity and relational dynamics in vector-borne disease risk

Tourism has yet to figure prominently in studies of MBD but epidemiologists, urban ecologists, and specialists in public health increasingly argue for more nuanced analyses of social complexity and relational dynamics in vector-borne disease risk. What are known as comprehensive 'social-ecological' frameworks have gained traction, moving beyond exclusively biological or physical explanations and challenging traditional, linear, and individually focused understandings of how diseases spread (Pickett et al., 2020). For example, Pickett et al. (2020: 305) argue that a conceptualisation of social complexity must transcend matters of human population density and aggregate demographic data, explicitly examining the roles of institutions, norms, social identity and status, as well as people's lifestyles and environmental interactions. By emphasising interfaces between wildlife and human populations, the influence of environmental conditions, and the roles of global trade and travel, approaches such as the One Health framework (Murray et al., 2022) locate transmission pathways within interdependent ecological domains rather than isolating human or viral factors. Such holistic frameworks recognise the need for incorporating multiple stakeholders, emphasising community engagement and culturally appropriate health education to empower communities in MBD control (Adnyana, 2024).

In this literature, the social components of human-mosquito interaction are situated within broader political, economic, and environmental contexts (Pickett et al. 2020). Rather than treating outbreaks as isolated events, the method is to frame epidemics as symptoms of systemic issues such as urban overcrowding, climate change, and inadequate sanitation, arguing that effective public health interventions must address 'structural' drivers. In addition, such approaches recognise that multiple, concurrent (syndemic) epidemics may interact with adverse social conditions such as poverty, marginalisation, and environmental degradation to amplify health burdens (Kelly, 2021).

Advances in computing and data science have paralleled and supported these conceptual shifts, expanding the capacity to measure complex interactions. The incorporation of computational social-science methods into epidemiology has demonstrated their value in capturing social domains, particularly behavioural heterogeneity and its relevance for the risk of exposure. Emerging data sources, including smartphone mobility records and environmental monitoring tools (e.g. Mosquito Citizen Science App reports, BG traps, AI-driven smart traps), now enable high-resolution modelling of the risk of mosquito-borne disease by linking human movement with environmental variables. As a result, researchers drawing on activity space and time-geography can map individuals' spatial and temporal activities, variation in social characteristics such as income, ethnicity, or occupation, mosquito exposure, and disease transmission with unprecedented precision (Citron et al., 2021).

These data-driven epidemiological approaches provide precise predictions of risk, but many continue to treat social and demographic factors as 'discrete, stable, homogeneous, and measurable' (Cohn, 2014: 157). While complex modelling depends on a wide range of inputs, analyses tend to prioritise individual behaviours or their aggregated representations. In other words, forms of methodological individualism persist in studies that correlate an ever-growing number of variables with increasingly marginal effects (Russo and Kelly, 2023).

One side effect is to obscure aspects of local variation. As Cohn notes, this is because modellers and epidemiologists 'pay little attention to power and sociality, and the emergent and contingent properties of people's *situated practices*' (2014: 157) (my italics). Writing of *Aedes*-borne viruses, Evans et al. (2021: 4) suggest that to effectively understand and address the fact that mosquito populations can be more abundant in either lower socio-economic neighbourhoods (LaDeau et al., 2013; Mulligan et al., 2015) or higher socio-economic areas (Becker et al., 2014; Mulligan et al., 2015), a place-based, integrative approach is needed, one that embeds ecological insights within their specific social contexts (Kinzig, 2001).

In what follows, I illustrate the salience of these conclusions with reference to tourist-related exposure to MBD in Catalonia, but before doing so, I discuss the relevance of multi-species analyses, and the contribution that practice theories can make to the field.

Multispecies and relational perspectives on urban disease ecology

Environmental political ecologists and critical geographers, along with scholars working in the environmental humanities, anthropology, and sociology continue to develop nuanced, relational and 'more-than-human' accounts of disease and exposure, all of which challenge conventional epidemiological models (see, for example, Wolf, 2016; Gandy, 2023; Shove et al., 2026).

Multispecies ethnographies have highlighted the entanglements of human and non-human lives within specific socio-political and ecological contexts (Kirksey and Helmreich, 2010; Rigby, 2018). For example, Beisel and Wergin (2022) show how mosquito mobilities are shaped by infrastructural and political processes across multiple sites (see also Robbins and Miller, 2013). Kelly and Lezaun's (2014) study of malaria control in Dar es Salaam is similar in that it treats mosquito management as an infrastructural and political practice and goes on to describe how mosquitoes adapt to urban rhythms and policy interventions. In various works Gandy (see for example 2019; 2022; 2023) takes much the same approach, explaining the proliferation of mosquito populations as a symptom of failing systems of governance and urbanisation.

In an article in which she argues for multiple analytical approaches, Meike Wolf (2016) conceptualises urban epidemics as 'biocultural phenomena' that emerge at the intersections of environmental conditions, microbial ecologies, and social practices. Amongst other things, Wolf emphasises the importance of understanding how infectious diseases manifest themselves differently in different local contexts. Drawing on comparative ethnographies, she argues that vulnerabilities vary dramatically with climate, infrastructure, governance, and cultural norms.

Despite relevant differences of focus and emphasis, all the authors mentioned above reject static or bounded notions of the city; instead, urban space is conceptualised as heterogeneous, relational, and continuously (re) produced through dynamic assemblages of ecological, social, political, infrastructural relations and multispecies entanglements.

This relational view connects local disease ecologies to global flows of capital, labour, and pathogens (Connolly et al., 2021; Hinchliffe, 2013), suggesting that infrastructures, pipes, waste channels, and patterns of informal housing create conditions for mosquito reproduction and human exposure (Beisel and Wergin, 2022; Gandy, 2023). Building on these ideas, epidemiology is understood not as a technical enterprise, but as an exercise in identifying multispecies urban assemblages shaped by histories of colonialism, capitalist development, and infrastructural politics (Robbins and Miller, 2013; Gandy 2023). According to Evans et al. (2022) this is also something of a problem. It is so in that social theories and sociological critiques resist easy quantification and rarely identify simple pathways toward actionable solutions (Russo and Kelly, 2023). This is especially true for authors who challenge the simplifications and spatial fixities on which public health interventions typically depend.

To reiterate, disease exposure and transmission are increasingly understood as more than just a 'three-species interaction problem'. There is widespread agreement that it is important to consider the role of multiple social factors, however conceived. In the next section I suggest that practice theories provide a means of bringing some of these dimensions together.

Conceptualising practices, materials and multispecies entanglements

Rather than focusing on individual choices, behaviours, or reified social structures, theorists like Giddens argue that practices represent the primary unit of social analysis (Giddens, 1984). Schatzki defines practices as 'embodied, materially mediated arrays of human activity centrally organised around shared practical understanding' (2001: 11). For Shove et al. (2012) practices consist of active integrations of materials, meanings and competences. As such they constitute socially shared patterns of activity (Watson and Shove, 2022: 5) that unfold temporally and spatially as configurations of doings and sayings (Schatzki, 1996), and that endure as recognisable 'blocks' realised through enactments by individuals and groups (Reckwitz, 2002). More than that, practices interconnect, giving rise to extensive complexes and configurations (Hui et al., 2017).

It is important to recognise that the ongoing integration of meanings, materials, and competences is inherently dynamic and that practices are continuously reproduced, adapted, or disrupted across sites. They are not necessarily habitual, and as Blue et al. (2016: 3) note, any one practice encompasses multiple possible performances. This fluidity is consistent with the relational approaches introduced above, but a focus on social practices arguably changes the focus and the frame of reference. In what follows I use aspects of practice theory's conceptual repertoire to develop a method of attending to human–mosquito interactions and MBD transmission. Using tourist practice as an example, I show how practice theory can be a 'heuristic aid' (Reckwitz, 2016) that helps foster interdisciplinary dialogue and empirical investigation.

In essence I argue that MBD transmission is shaped by the distributed, relational and recursive nature of practices that are always enacted as part of/ within distinct material (ecological) arrangements. Through their multi-sited and intersecting enactment, practices differentially mediate relations between humans, mosquitoes and environments, thereby shaping MBD risk across landscapes from the local to the transnational. This reconceptualisation builds on Shove et al.'s (2026) argument that the spread of infection depends on the multi-sited enactment of similar conjunctions of practices and the conditions and habitats associated with them. By foregrounding the heterogeneity of how practices are performed, and by recognising that practices are always on the move, I respond to Wolf's (2016) call to analyse the 'locally contingent' manifestations of infectious disease, and to describe what Hinchliffe et al. refer to as 'disease situations' (Hinchliffe et al, 2017: XV) (see also Shove, Chapter 2).

Tourist practices and exposure to mosquito-borne disease

There is a significant literature on the history of tourism, and the practices associated with it. Rather than going back in time, I focus on the experiences of a handful of tourists in Barcelona today. These few experiences underline the different forms that 'tourist practices' take, and their uneven reproduction across local, regional, national, and international scales. This includes the consistent or inconsistent performance of practices related to mosquito exposure, habitat formation and disease mitigation (health practices) in different settings. Of course, tourism (De Souza Bispo, 2016; Lamers et al., 2017) is only one form of human movement: others include migration, education, and forced displacement. In all these examples, and more, analysing which practices are carried over (Maller and Strengers, 2013) or re-enacted in new contexts helps to explain exposure and transmission in ways that move beyond common emphases on the cultural or ethnic representation of mobile bodies.

Observations and interviews with tourists in Ciutadella Park, Barcelona provide some insight into forms of exposure associated with tourism, and more specifically with practices such as sunbathing, yoga and socialising. As described, variations in vulnerability map on to the different ways in which these practices are enacted in similar environmental settings.

The first example concerns Jenny (pseudonyms are used throughout), a visitor from the UK attending a yoga workshop organised around concepts of relaxation, self-development and social connection. The materials involved included a blanket, yoga mat, book, food and a reusable water bottle along with the park's lawns, trees and ornamental features that afforded shade and space for stretching. Jenny's risk of exposure was increased because of her focus on yoga practice (being barefoot, not using insect repellent for example), rather than mosquito avoidance. By contrast, Sara, a tourist from the United States, enjoyed the same space (lawns, scattered tree cover, open space), but she used insect repellent in part because of prior experience in Florida, where mosquitoes are ubiquitous. Sarah did not view Barcelona as 'high-risk' for mosquito-borne disease, but her 'embodied knowledge' and reproduction of past 'health practices' mitigated exposure.

Jenny and Sara's tourist practices took place in the same park, the vegetation of which can also provide habitats for mosquitoes. Both women associated the park with leisure and relaxation but in privileging bodily freedom (Jenny), or routinised bodily care (Sara), their practices generated different forms of vulnerability. As represented here, the material arrangements of Ciutadella Park are integral to the formation of human–mosquito interactions. As described, the park is a space in which leisure practices such as yoga, sunbathing and socialising take place and a habitat that can sustain mosquito populations. In this respect, the park constitutes what I describe as multiple and fluid geographies of exposure.

Tourism and the geographies of exposure

Schatzki's (2010) site ontology provides a way of theorising the spatial distribution of practices, conceiving of the social as a metaphorical site in which practices and material arrangements hang together. Within this ontology, *places* are localised 'doings-places' anchored at objects where practices unfold (Hui and Walker, 2018). Places are connected by paths (defined by embodied movements like those associated with practices of mobility), and *settings* are the wider arrangements that integrate multiple places and paths into broader fields of activity. These dimensions are not external containers (contexts) for action but integral to its very constitution. In other words, practices do not simply occur *in* places and settings but actively take shape *through* them.

This perspective is particularly useful for studying human–mosquito interactions in which the spatial choreography of practices intersects with ecological affordances to produce differential risks of exposure. As Hui and Walker (2018) explain, it is important to note that the spatialities of practices are meaningful in that they are shaped by goals/ends, and connected in ways that activity space, and time-geography approaches do not capture.

By way of illustration, it is useful to consider some of the practices Jenny enacts over the course of her day. This begins in her hotel room, already a setting of potential exposure. A bed functions as a place for sleeping, relaxing or reading, but it can also become a place in which mosquitoes bite (especially from mosquitoes that bite at night such as the *Culex* mosquito), depending on the configuration of other material arrangements including windows and air conditioning. As this example suggests, the design of the hotel room shows how practices and arrangements hang together (Schatzki, 2002), simultaneously affording comfort and producing conditions of vulnerability.

Later, Jenny joins her companions for a yoga session at the Greek Amphitheatre in Montjuïc Park. Here, the amphitheatre's stone tiers and surrounding vegetation are not mere backdrops but integral elements of a practice-arrangement bundle that makes yoga both possible and meaningful. The aesthetic qualities of stone and greenery reflect cultural concepts of nature and beauty, while at the same time providing shaded niches and plants amongst which mosquitoes live. In this setting, the same material arrangements generate the affordances of human practice and the conditions of exposure. From the amphitheatre, Jenny wanders through the wider Montjuïc area, stops for lunch at a local bar, and eventually travels along city streets toward Ciutadella Park. This movement is not a simple transfer between destinations, but a path composed of successive segments of green spaces, shaded underpasses, and busy plazas, each with its own ecological affordances and each a point at which Jenny's path can intersect with the paths of mosquitoes – creating conditions of (potential) exposure.

Joanna, a visitor from Washington, D.C., follows a different route: one that includes Montjuïc Castle, Tibidabo's Sagrat Cor Church and its surrounding greenbelt, and finally Ciutadella Park. Her movements link multiple settings and places, drawing together architectural landmarks, forested tracts, and urban infrastructures.

As these cases show, walking, cycling and using public transport are associated with distinct *paths*: a shaded trail, a cycle lane, a crowded bus route. These are not inert conduits but routes that incorporate and depend upon distinct material arrangements and ecological conditions. As with Sara, Joanna's prior experiences with mosquitoes at home and on other trips mean that she applies insect repellent as a matter of course. In effect health practices (like using repellent) are woven into the same practice-arrangement bundles that connect leisure, mobility and ecological exposure.

Tourism and the timing of exposure

The timing of practices is as significant as their spatial arrangement when it comes to human-mosquito interaction. *Aedes albopictus,* for example, is most active at dawn and dusk, while *Culex* tends to bite at night. This means that seemingly benign practices, such as resting, cooling the body, or early morning exercise, are epidemiologically relevant because of when they occur. As Blue notes, 'in reproducing social life, practices are repeated in sequences and combinations that exhibit various forms of temporal connection' (Blue, 2019: 2).

Although tourism is often described as an 'escape attempt' from the structures of everyday life (Cohen and Taylor, 2003), tourist practices reproduce temporal patterns shaped by, amongst other things, the timing and duration of vacations, attraction opening hours, transport timetables, mealtimes (including siesta), weather conditions and the timespaces of other practitioners. This is important in that, the 'where' of a practice is always bound up with a 'when', and vice versa. For instance, Jenny's yoga practice in Montjuïc is not only located in the amphitheatre gardens but it involves the co-presence of fellow yoga practitioners and is scheduled for sunrise. It is this timespace, 'Montjuïc-at-sunrise' that constitutes both a meaningful setting for her practice (quiet, cool, tranquil, natural) and a heightened risk of exposure in that it coincides with peak mosquito activity.

Practices rarely occur in isolation; rather, they synchronise around shared timespaces. The Barcelona Zoo, located in Ciutadella Park, and also known for the presence of mosquitoes, is a good example. The zoo is open from 10 am to 8 pm and is visited by large numbers of tourists and residents. The timespaces of the zoo are made by diverse practices such as visiting, observing, strolling, eating and resting. When these coincide with the timespaces of mosquitoes, the likelihood of risky encounters increases.

Connecting humans and mosquitoes

In combination, these brief examples show how practices and material arrangements bring humans and mosquitoes together across time and space, creating opportunities for human-mosquito interaction and MBD transmission. These connections happen as a result of multiple aspects of practice including: (1) constitutive meanings, such as a 'good holiday', 'exploration' or 'self-development'; (2) overlapping material arrangements and infrastructures that are integral to or that afford and stabilise practice; (3) competences and shared bodily performances that carry across sites; (4) forms of temporal coordination and (5) environments in which tiger mosquitoes live. Together, these aspects link visitors, local residents, and mosquito habitats, producing shifting and variable pathways of exposure.

When practitioners move across or through sites, they carry or enact practices shaped and connected by shared meanings and motivations. Jenny's yoga practices, for instance, are linked by values of health, well-being and discovery, connecting her to fellow practitioners and to mosquito habitats. This is not a static configuration and encounters with mosquitoes, through bites or illness, can alter perceptions of risk in space and time. Again, there is no consistent pattern. For example, one participant explained that severe reactions to bites in Athens led him to adopt protective routines (repellent, clothing, air-conditioning) in different settings, including Barcelona. By contrast, a participant who had previously experienced dengue infection in Colombia took little or no account of the risk in Barcelona. For practice theorists, such variability is a reminder of the fact that meanings and actions are embedded in or constituted by differing social-material arrangements in ways that compromise theories of individual choice, value and rational action.

Materials, infrastructures and exposure: How infections spread

As touched upon above, materials and infrastructures connect practices, practitioners and multispecies ecologies across geographical space. In the examples I have discussed, they stabilise and coordinate practices (Shove, 2017) while simultaneously bringing humans into proximity with mosquitoes.

Transport infrastructures, for instance, channel encounters with specific species and link otherwise separate ecological niches. Long-distance transportation systems (planes, trains, buses) extend this connectivity globally, moving humans, mosquitoes and pathogens across ecological zones. The globalisation of *Aedes albopictus* consequently reflects not just trade infrastructures but the embodied enactment of practices that animate them. In other words, infrastructures do not simply provide static risk factors; their entanglement in multiple practices actively sustains some pathways of exposure and not others. From this perspective, disease transmission is not localised in isolated hotspots, but is continuously (re)produced through relational spatial dynamics of practices that extend across urban landscapes and the more-than-human encounters they help shape.

In this analysis, defensive practices like correctly applying insect repellent, wearing long-sleeved clothing or recognising high-risk environments, also unfold within social and material contexts. As described above, these arrangements can travel with individual practitioners and take hold in new environments. This is important in that practices like those of yoga or sightseeing are not simply replicated in different settings but are reconfigured alongside material arrangements, infrastructures, and spatial and temporal conventions (Maller and Strengers, 2013).

This is relevant in that understanding which practices circulate (and which do not) is essential in understanding how human exposure to mosquitoes arises. However, this is only part of the story. As described, the geographies of human-mosquito interaction and mosquito-borne disease transmission emerge from the repeated enactment of constellations of practices across diverse sites. To be precise, transmission only occurs when practices unfold within or as part of particular material-ecological assemblages.

In summary, material arrangements both enable and constrain action, channelling and prefiguring the spatial and temporal dynamics of practices and the habitats in which mosquitoes thrive. Features such as housing design, public plazas, shelters, weather conditions, shade and greenery not only figure within and as part of human practices, but they also constitute ecological niches that shape the distribution of mosquitoes and their behaviour. Sources of blood meals, including human bodies, are integral to these niches but as I have also pointed out, this relationship is reciprocal. It is so in that the presence of mosquitoes such as *Aedes albopictus* prompts people to avoid certain areas, to use repellents and nets, or to develop technologies and tools that can help track insect populations.

As emphasised at the outset microbial parasites remain ever present in this dance of human and non-human interaction. To reiterate, conditions of exposure do not stem from isolated environmental factors or discrete human activities, but from their ongoing, spatially and temporally dispersed entanglement. In other words, practices continually reproduce socio-ecological environments that sustain (or undermine) mosquito populations and arbovirus transmission. Further still, it is important to consider the role of other practices, including those of mosquito control (removing of stagnant water receptacles, fumigation, adaptation of drainage infrastructure and even the choice of greenery).

Methodological and practical implications

In this final section I comment on the methodological implications of these ideas. Understanding the intermingling of human and non-human entities (including mosquitoes and infections) arguably depends on understanding how practices change and spread over time and space.

This calls for a reorientation in how existing methods and data are conceptualised. Spatial and mobility-based approaches – such as activity-space analysis, time-space paths, Geographical Information System (GIS) and Global Positioning System (GPS) tracking – are widely used to map exposure, yet typically rest on assumptions of objective space, individual movement and environmental risk, offering limited insight into the practices enacted within these spaces, including shared ends, competences, materials and their linkage across sites and times. From a practice perspective, spatial traces should therefore be treated not as direct indicators of exposure but as partial expressions of interwoven practice performances unfolding in space and time, requiring practice-sensitive enquiry (e.g. qualitative GIS, interviews, diaries, and map-based elicitation) capable of situating movement within broader bundles of practices. In contrast to behavioural or risk-factor models that isolate variables or posit linear determinants, a practice-oriented approach conceptualises exposure as an emergent property of dynamically related practice elements and socio-material arrangements, such that changes in materials, competences, shared ends, or wider arrangements (including climatic conditions) generate spatially and temporally uneven effects. Combined with entomological, meteorological and socio-demographic data, this approach argues for methods of tracing multispecies, multi-sited entanglements and for shifting analysis away from variable-based explanation toward understanding how configurations of practices produce mosquito–human interaction and disease risk. At the same time, this reorientation entails limits: as Cohn (2014) argues, complexity-oriented approaches offer only partial and situated interpretations, and a focus on practices does not yield simple or linear prescriptions for intervention (Blue et al., 2016). Instead, there is a need for more reflexive, adaptive and context-sensitive public health engagement amid ongoing ontological and translational tensions (Southerton and Whillans, 2024).

A second, complementary route depends on developing historical accounts of how present geographies of mosquitoes and diseases have been shaped by past and ongoing complexes of practices and material arrangements. This might involve the careful production of situated histories of practices that intersect and/or influence mosquito attraction and repellence. Research along these lines would help understand the emergence of mosquito microbiomes and of the practices that shape them, including local histories of biofilms and communities of microorganisms in breeding sites (such as those found on stagnant water), or in situations that provide essential food sources and influence larval development. Such an approach would be in line with that proposed by Shove (Chapter 2) and would include historical accounts of the stability and mobility of human populations and the 'disease situations' associated with practice differentiated ways of life, such as the diverse forms of tourism as touched upon above.

In conclusion, and as this chapter suggests, focusing on social practice (not on human behaviour, and not on ecological systems in isolation) calls for creative methodologies, attuned to the recursive, dynamic entanglements through which urban ecologies and disease pathways are continually reproduced. Taking up these challenges requires interdisciplinary collaboration, methodological flexibility and theoretical sensitivity to the sorts of questions that are, and are not, compatible with a focus on social practices as these constitute forms of health, exposure and multispecies life.

References

Adnyana, I.M.D.M. (2024). 'The imperative of a comprehensive One Health approach for mosquito-borne disease control in Indonesia', *Qeios*: 1–11. https://doi.org/10.32388/6JT36Y.

Becker, B., Leisnham, P.T. and LaDeau, S.L. (2014). 'A tale of two city blocks: differences in immature and adult mosquito abundances between socioeconomically different urban blocks in Baltimore (Maryland, USA)', *International Journal of Environmental Research and Public Health,* 11(3): 3256–3270. https://doi.org/10.3390/ijerph110303256.

Beisel, U. and Wergin, C. (2022). 'Understanding multispecies mobilities: from mosquito eradication to coexistence' in Hall, M. and Tamïr, D. (eds.) *Mosquitopia: the place of pests in a healthy world.* New York: Routledge. 32–46. https://doi.org/10.4324/9781003056034-4.

Biehler, D., Leisnham, P.T., LaDeau, S.L. and Bodner, D. (2019). 'Knowing nature and community through mosquitoes: reframing pest management through lay vector ecologies', *Local Environment*, 24(12): 1119–1135. https://doi.org/10.1080/13549839.2019.1681387.

Blue, S. (2019). 'Institutional rhythms: combining practice theory and rhythmanalysis to conceptualise processes of institutionalisation', *Time and Society*, 28(3): 922–950. https://doi.org/10.1177/0961463X17702165.

Blue, S., Shove, E., Carmona, C. and Kelly, M.P. (2016). 'Theories of practice and public health: understanding (un)healthy practices', *Critical Public Health*, 26(1): 36–50. https://doi.org/10.1080/09581596.2014.980396.

Citron, D.T., Iyer, S., Reiner, R.C. and Smith, D.L. (2021). 'Activity space maps: a novel human mobility data set for quantifying time spent at risk', *medRxiv*. https://doi.org/10.1101/2021.08.01.21261352.

Cohen, S. and Taylor, L. (2003). *Escape Attempts: The theory and practice of resistance in everyday life*. London: Routledge.

Cohn, S. (2014). 'From health behaviours to health practices' in Cohn, S. (ed) *From health behaviours to health practices: critical perspectives*. Chichester: Wiley Blackwell. 1–6. https://doi.org/10.1002/9781118898345.ch1.

Connolly, C., Keil, R. and Ali, S.H. (2021). 'Extended urbanisation and the spatialities of infectious disease: demographic change, infrastructure and governance', *Urban Studies,* 58(2): 245–263. https://doi.org/10.1177/0042098020910873.

de Souza Bispo, M. (2016). 'Tourism as practice', *Annals of Tourism Research,* 61(1): 170–179. https://doi.org/10.1016/j.annals.2016.10.009.

Evans, M., Bhatnagar, S., Drake, J., Murdock, C. and Mukherjee, S. (2021). 'An integrative approach to mosquito dynamics reveals differences in people's everyday experiences of mosquitoes', *bioRxiv*. https://doi.org/10.1101/2021.09.06.459057.

Evans, M., Bhatnagar, S., Drake, J.M., Murdock, C.C. and Mukherjee, S. (2022). 'Socio-ecological dynamics in urban systems: an integrative approach to mosquito-borne disease in Bengaluru, India', *People and Nature*, 4(3): 730–743. https://doi.org/10.1002/pan3.10311.

Gandy, M. (2019). 'The fly that tried to save the world: saproxylic geographies and other-than-human ecologies', *Transactions of the Institute of British Geographers*, 44(2): 392–406. https://doi.org/10.1111/tran.12281.

Gandy, M. (2022). 'The zoonotic city: urban political ecology and the pandemic imaginary'. *International Journal of Urban and Regional Research*, 46(2): 202–219. https://doi.org/10.1111/1468-2427.13080.

Gandy, M. (2023). 'Zoonotic urbanisation: multispecies urbanism and the rescaling of urban epidemiology', *Urban Studies*, 60(13): 2529–2549. https://doi.org/10.1177/00420980231154802.

García-San-Miguel, L., Giménez-Durán, J., Saravia-Campelli, G., Calvo-Reyes, M.C., Fernández-Martínez, B., Frank, C., Wilking, H., Janer, R.G., Miranda, M.Á., Cano, E.A. and Moros, M.J.S. (2024). 'Detection of dengue in German tourists returning from Ibiza, Spain, related to an autochthonous outbreak, August to October 2022', *Eurosurveillance*, 29(14): 2300296. https://doi.org/10.2807/1560-7917.ES.2024.29.14.2300296.

Giddens, A. (1984). *The Constitution of Society: Outline of the theory of structuration*. Cambridge: Polity Press.

Gössling, S. (2002). 'Global environmental consequences of tourism', *Global Environmental Change*, 12(4): 283–302. https://doi.org/10.1016/S0959-3780(02)00044-4.

Herrero-Martínez, J.M., Sánchez-Ledesma, M. and Ramos-Rincón, J.M. (2023). 'Imported and autochthonous dengue in Spain', *Revista Clínica Española*, 223(8): 510–519. https://doi.org/10.1016/j.rceng.2023.07.007.

Hinchliffe, S. (2013). 'The insecurity of biosecurity: remaking emerging infectious diseases' in Dobson, A., Barker, K. and Taylor, S.L. (eds.) *Biosecurity: the socio-politics of invasive species and infectious diseases*. London: Routledge. 199–213.

Hinchliffe, S., Bingham, N., Allen, J. and Carter, S. (2017). *Pathological Lives: Disease, space and biopolitics*. Chichester: Wiley.

Hinchliffe, S., Bingham, N., Allen, J. and Carter, S. (2017). *Pathological Lives: Disease, space and biopolitics*. Chichester: Wiley.

Hui, A., Schatzki, T. and Shove, E. (eds.) (2017). *The Nexus of Practices: Connections, constellations, practitioners*. London: Routledge. https://doi.org/10.4324/9781315560816.

Hui, A. and Walker, G. (2018). 'Concepts and methodologies for a new relational geography of energy demand: social practices, doing-places and settings', *Energy Research and Social Science*, 39: 39–50. https://doi.org/10.1016/j.erss.2017.09.032.

Kelly, A.H. and Lezaun, J. (2014). 'Urban mosquitoes, situational publics, and the pursuit of interspecies separation in Dar es Salaam', *American Ethnologist*, 41(2): 368–383. https://doi.org/10.1111/amet.12081.

Kelly, M.P. (2021). 'The relation between the social and the biological and COVID-19', *Public Health*, 196: 18–23. https://doi.org/10.1016/j.puhe.2021.05.003.

Kinzig, A.P. (2001). 'Bridging disciplinary divides to address environmental and intellectual challenges', *Ecosystems*, 4(8): 709–715. https://doi.org/10.1007/s10021-001-0039-7.

Kirksey, S. and Helmreich, S. (2010) 'The emergence of multispecies ethnography'. *Cultural Anthropology*, 25(4), 545–576. https://doi.org/10.1111/j.1548-1360.2010.01069.x

LaDeau, S.L., Leisnham, P.T., Biehler, D. and Bodner, D. (2013). 'Higher mosquito production in low-income neighborhoods of Baltimore and Washington, DC: understanding ecological drivers and mosquito-borne disease risk in temperate cities', *International Journal of Environmental Research and Public Health*, 10(4): 1505–1526. https://doi.org/10.3390/ijerph10041505.

Lamers, M., van der Duim, R. and Spaargaren, G. (2017). 'The relevance of practice theories for tourism research', *Annals of Tourism Research*, 62(1): 54–63. https://doi.org/10.1016/j.annals.2016.12.002.

Maller, C. and Strengers, Y. (2013). 'The global migration of everyday life: investigating the practice memories of Australian migrants', *Geoforum*, 44(1): 243–252. https://doi.org/10.1016/j.geoforum.2012.09.002.

Michalet, S., Minard, G., Chevalier, W., Meiffren, G., Saucereau, Y., Tran Van, V., Comte, G., Tran, F.H. and Valiente Moro, C. (2019). 'Identification of human skin bacteria attractive to the Asian tiger mosquito', *Environmental Microbiology*, 21(12): 4662–4674. https://doi.org/10.1111/1462-2920.14793.

Mulligan, K., Dixon, J., Sinn, C.-L.J. and Elliott, S.J. (2015). 'Is dengue a disease of poverty? A systematic review', *Pathogens and Global Health*, 109(1): 10–18. https://doi.org/10.1179/2047773214Y.0000000168.

Murray, M.H., Buckley, J., Byers, K.A., Fake, K., Lehrer, E.W., Magle, S.B., Stone, C., Tuten, H. and Schell, C.J. (2022). 'One health for all: advancing human and ecosystem health in cities by integrating an environmental justice lens', *Annual Review of Ecology, Evolution, and Systematics*, 53: 403–426. https://doi.org/10.1146/annurev-ecolsys-102220-031745.

Pickering, A. (1995). *The Mangle of Practice: Time, agency, and science*. Chicago: University of Chicago Press. https://doi.org/10.7208/chicago/9780226668253.001.0001.

Pickett, S.T.A., Cadenasso, M.L., Baker, M.E., Band, L.E., Boone, C.G., Buckley, G.L., Groffman, P.M., Grove, J.M., Irwin, E.G., Kaushal, S.S., LaDeau, S.L., Miller, A.J., Nilon, C.H., Romolini, M., Rosi, E.J., Swan, C.M. and Szlavecz, K. (2020). 'Theoretical perspectives of the Baltimore ecosystem study: conceptual evolution in a social–ecological research project', *BioScience*, 70(4): 297–314. https://doi.org/10.1093/biosci/biz166.

Powell, J.R. (2019). 'An evolutionary perspective on vector-borne diseases', *Frontiers in Genetics*, 10: 1266. https://doi.org/10.3389/fgene.2019.01266.

Reckwitz, A. (2002). 'Toward a theory of social practices: a development in culturalist theorizing', *European Journal of Social Theory*, 5(2): 243–263. https://doi.org/10.1177/13684310222225432.

Reckwitz, A. (2016). 'Practices and their affects' in Hui, A., Schatzki, T. and Shove, E. (eds.) *The Nexus of Practices: Connections, constellations, practitioners*. London: Routledge. 144–158. https://doi.org/10.4324/9781315560816.

Rigby, K. (2018). 'Feathering the multispecies nest: green cities, convivial spaces', *RCC Perspectives*, 1: 73–80. doi.org/10.5282/rcc/8469.

Robbins, P. and Miller, J.C. (2013). 'The mosquito state: how technology, capital, and state practice mediate the ecologies of public health' in King, B. and Crews, K. (eds.) *Ecologies and politics of health*. London: Routledge. 196–216. https://doi.org/10.4324/9780203115527.

Rose, N.H., Sylla, M., Badolo, A., Lutomiah, J., Ayala, D., Aribodor, O.B., Ibe, N., Akorli, J., Otoo, S., Mutebi, J.P. and Kriete, A.L. (2020). 'Climate and urbanization drive mosquito preference for humans', *Current Biology*, 30(18): 3570–3579. https://doi.org/10.1016/j.cub.2020.06.092.

Russo, F. and Kelly, M.P. (2023). 'The "lifeworld" of health and disease and the design of public health interventions', *Longitudinal and Life Course Studies*, 15(1): 25–44. https://doi.org/10.1332/175795921X16835353334712.

Schatzki, T. (1996). *Social Practices: A Wittgensteinian approach to human activity and the social*. Cambridge: Cambridge University Press. https://doi.org/10.1017/CBO9780511527470.

Schatzki, T. (2002). *The Site of the Social: A philosophical account of the constitution of social life and change*. Pennsylvania State University Press: University Park, PA.

Schatzki, T. (2010). *The Timespace of Human Activity: On performance, society, and history as indeterminate teleological events*. Lanham: Lexington Books. https://doi.org/10.5040/9781978737358.

Schatzki, T., Knorr-Cetina, K. and Von Savigny, E. (eds.) (2001). *The Practice Turn in Contemporary Theory*. London: Routledge. https://doi.org/10.4324/9780203977453.

Shirai, Y., Funada, H., Takizawa, H., Seki, T., Morohashi, M. and Kamimura, K., (2004) 'Landing Preference of Aedes albopictus (Diptera: Culicidae) on Human Skin Among ABO Blood Groups, Secretors or Nonsecretors, and ABH Antigens' *Journal of Medical Entomology*, 41 (4): 796–799, https://doi.org/10.1603/0022-2585-41.4.796

Shove, E. (2017). 'Matters of practice' in Hui, A., Schatzki, T. and Shove, E. (eds.) *The Nexus of Practices: Connections, constellations, practitioners*. London: Routledge. https://doi.org/10.4324/9781315560816.

Shove, E., Blue, S. and Kelly, M.P. (2026). *Practice Theory and the Biosocial: Microbes, matter and milieu*. Oxford: Berghahn. https://doi.org/10.3167/9781836953395

Shove, E., Pantzar, M. and Watson, M. (2012). *The Dynamics of Social Practice: Everyday life and how it changes*. London: Sage. https://doi.org/10.4135/9781446250655.

Southerton, D. and Whillans, J. (2024). 'Time use surveys, social practice theory, and activity connections', *The British Journal of Sociology*, 75(2): 168–186. https://doi.org/10.1111/1468-4446.13073.

Watson, M. and Shove, E. (2022). How infrastructures and practices shape each other: aggregation, integration and the introduction of gas central heating. *Sociological Research Online*. January 2022. doi:10.1177/13607804211055495

Willoughby, J.R., McKenzie, B.A., Ahn, J., Steury, T.D., Lepczyk, C.A. and Zohdy, S. (2022). 'Mosquito invasion via the global shipping network is slowed in high-risk areas by on-shore and ship-board monitoring', *bioRxiv*. https://doi.org/10.1101/2022.08.29.505734.

Wolf, M. (2016). 'Rethinking urban epidemiology: natures, networks and materialities', *International Journal of Urban and Regional Research*, 40(5): 958–982. https://doi.org/10.1111/1468-2427.12381.

PART II

Framing matters of microscopic materiality

Cecily Maller

This part of the book considers microscopic materiality and how it is represented in social theories along with ideas about how to change human-microbial relations in a series of different practices, products and settings in agriculture, urban environments and inside buildings. On the surface, the four chapters in this section are all quite different. Maller is interested in how microbes are represented in theories of practice. Cusworth and colleagues critique the practices of modern agriculture which have reduced the ability of the soil microbiome to support crop fertility and immunity to disease. Brown and co-authors discuss the architecture and design of hospitals in illness prevention and treatment while Jauho explores allergy prevention in Finland. Considering these different foci, what the chapters share is an interest in the material effects of microbes, microbiomes and other microscopic entities in and on bodies, plants, air, soil (including allergens and agricultural chemicals) and the biosocial flows through and comprising various practices, and how different ways of understanding microbial relationships and their effects could reframe interventions to tackle complex agricultural, human and animal health problems. Although they draw on different conceptualisations of practices, including how they come into being and are reproduced, these propositions collectively place microbes and their material effects at the centre of the topics being investigated. As a set, the chapters are also linked by an interest in the changing conditions of encounter in built and outdoor environments, and how microbes could more generally be enrolled in achieving balanced states of health.

Maller opens this section by exploring how materiality is generally conceived of in theories of social practice and how social practice theory can reframe everyday relations with microbes and microbiomes in various

DOI: 10.4324/9781003685210-5

settings. She discusses how microbes and microbial ecologies are represented in social practices, taking into consideration the possibility that they could be seen as types of materials and performers of practice. The specific theorisation may be dependent on the relevant human-microbial relations at play, the practices of empirical concern, and the questions that need answers in any given place and time. But to avoid analyses that focus on people, microbes or some other entity and detracting from the agency of practices, she arrives at the notion that microbes are part of the biosocial that flows through and comprise practices, along with many other sorts of materialities. Maller reminds readers that seeing the world through practices rather than in terms of seemingly problematic entities or outcomes, such as a single disease or organism, leads to different ways of understanding problems or designing interventions to tackle them, a key aim of this collection.

In her discussion, Maller also tackles entrenched notions of antimicrobial sentiment. She explains that despite common assumptions, most microbes are generally beneficial or at least are not harmful. However, antimicrobial views about microbes tend to dominate health and cleanliness discourses, perpetuating negative meanings that may be causing more harm than good. She discusses how narratives of antimicrobiality could be reframed to be affirmative, adaptive and probiotic heading towards a form of post-Pasteurian stewardship.

The next three chapters also centre on microscopic materiality and relationality, focusing on the sites of interaction or intervention (or where and how humans and non-humans interact) and the effects of practices on people, environments and microbes. Although this approach might differ from other chapters that begin with a deeper anchoring in social practice theory, the arguments and examples seek to challenge conventional approaches to understanding disease and ill health through the isolated study of the behaviour of people or microbes, decontextualised from socio-material and historical relations.

Looking at the effects of practices of the past, Cusworth and colleagues turn their attention to agriculture, beginning with a critique of modern techniques which have undermined the ability of the soil microbiome to support the production of healthy and sufficient food crops. They start by explaining that in reducing the diversity of soil microbiomes, widespread antimicrobial manipulation means that soils become less fertile and that crops become less resistant to disease. In a cascading effect, the loss of soil functionality increases reliance on harmful practices that use chemicals and fertilisers to produce sufficient crop yields. Cusworth et al. show that the overuse of antimicrobial drugs has unbalanced agricultural systems, which not only causes dysbiosis (microbial dysfunction), but has other unintended consequences. Highlighting the complex spatiotemporal relations of agricultural practices, another effect is the creation of resistant strains of bacteria that travel from farms to human bodies and other environments, contributing to the diffusion of antimicrobial resistance (AMR) and highlighting the porosity of bodies and barriers.

The authors propose practices of 'microbial repair' as a way of changing course and reducing encounters with resistant microbes, while also encouraging soil health and other benefits. Envisioning this move through 'biosocial farming practices', they propose three sets of practices coming under the notion of microbial repair: attunement, co-cultivation and collective care. Through taking an agroecological approach, they make visible previously hidden relations between microbes, animals and people responsible for the production, decomposition, circulation and wider metabolisms in soils and on farms, drawing on a series of examples of UK-based agricultural production. Like Maller, they propose an affirmative or post-Pasteurian approach to human-microbial relations that involves a recalibration of pervasive antibiotic models.

The chapter led by Brown et al. connects with the previous two chapters but in a very different setting and from a different theoretical starting point. These authors focus on contrasting 'architectural dispositifs' in periods before and since the introduction of antibiotics in the 1940s and 1950s and explore healthcare buildings as materially-discursive expressions of human-microbial co-evolution. An 'architectural dispositif' is defined as the way human-microbial and other material relations are conceptualised, reconfigured and physically manifested in heterogeneous ensembles, such as a hospital.

Presenting a potted history of ideas about human-microbial relations and the risks of infection and approaches to treatment, they discuss three exemplar dispositifs over different eras to illustrate how air, microbes and hospitals intersect. In these examples, they concentrate on the effects of practices and the sorts of exchanges and outcomes they facilitate. The first example is the Papworth tuberculosis settlement outside Cambridge, UK, established in 1917. In this case, Brown et al. explore the design and use of outdoor huts and dwellings to house infectious patients in continuous, open-air 'aerotherapeutic' conditions. The second dispositif is a multi-storey hospital that opened in the late 1970s in a provincial northern British city and that relied on antibiotic approaches. The third is an infectious diseases hospital built in the mid-2000s in Sweden with an explicit brief to cater for a 'post-antibiotic future'. For each example they use archival historical and secondary sources and fieldwork comprising interviews, site visits and observations.

They connect with the previous chapters in sharing a critique of blunt antimicrobial approaches that seek to control, protect and manage human-microbial relations in-situ. Focusing on air rather than soil, like Cusworth and colleagues, Brown et al. discuss the intangibility and illegibility of air as an invisible medium, but as one that must be managed in healthcare settings. For example, they discuss the circulation of 'fresh' outdoor aerobiomes into clinical and other settings and the rearrangement of the built form to partially separate treatment spaces from those of administration. As with other chapters, the method is to follow 'biosocial' flows to illustrate the permeability of bodies and buildings, and how this can be disrupted by technologies and design with unintended consequences.

Brown et al. also deal with the downstream end of AMR in clinical settings, connecting with Cusworth et al. who discuss some of the practices in which AMR originates. In this case, the aim is to describe how an over-reliance on antibiotic measures that enclosed patients in crowded, sealed, urban conditions backfired with the emergence of AMR, prompting reconsideration of 'antibiotic' hospital architectures.

Taking practices as the conceptual starting point encourages broader socio-historical and socio-material exploration of flows, connecting complexes and bundles of practices that could explain the generation of problems like those of AMR. Brown et al. consequently propose that healthcare practices maintain a connection to historical ideas about beneficial human-microbial relations and healthy encounters in healthcare environments, while also remaining open to uncertain futures. This stance recognises that practices and their material arrangements are in a constant state of flux and flow and their trajectories cannot necessarily be easily controlled or directed towards certain outcomes.

The final chapter in this section by Jauho, although different in approach and emphasis, also picks up on some of the themes of previous chapters that foreground human-microbial relations and the effects of practices. Geographically, the chapter focuses on Finland and state initiatives to address rising cases of allergy and autoimmune conditions using affirmative microbial interventions. Underlying this interest is a concern about the reduction in exposure to microbially rich environments through the life course that can boost the immune system function. Jauho introduces the idea of 'holobiont public health' which views health as a multispecies or multi-relational achievement. Taking in medical and everyday interventions, similar to Brown et al., he reviews the Finnish National Allergy Program (2008–2018) and the Finnish Allergy, Skin, and Asthma Federation's National Nature Health Program (2023–2026), among others, which attempt to steer ideas about microbes and allergens from risk and avoidance of allergens to 'healthy' encounters based on the biodiversity hypothesis.

In discussing these programmes, Jauho is interested in using theories of social practice to help conceptualise human-microbial relations and interventions to address and evaluate them. This chapter also presents criticisms of the usual approaches to treat health and illness, in this case allergies, that have not been as successful as hoped and have had perverse or unexpected consequences. For allergies, dominant strategies are based on avoidance, medication, alleviation of symptoms and immunotherapy to desensitise bodies through controlled exposure, rather than on the ongoing intermingling of humans and microbes. Some of the interventions described are highly novel and involve substituting elements of practices or changing their materiality. For example, new products such as landscaping materials have been designed to ensure children are exposed to 'beneficial' and diverse microbes when engaging in outdoor play. Others include patented microbial extracts, dusts and powders which can potentially be added to common products in homes to provide regular, controlled beneficial microbial contact through everyday practices. A second set of examples has to do with the material infrastructure of environments such as urban green areas, redesigned to increase microbial encounters. Like other authors who consider scenarios in which human-microbial relations occur and encounters happen, Jauho writes about how various practices interact and how these interactions could be the target of future public health interventions.

In conclusion, this set of chapters, although not evenly arising from practice theoretical framings, consistently adopt hybrid biological and social approaches to human-microbial relations that account for histories, materialities and other forms of interaction and encounter. In their own ways they show that microbes are neither inherently good nor bad, and that alternative methods of managing the prevention and treatment of disease, or of maintaining and repairing ecosystems, are required to tackle some of the problems the world is now facing. Informed by theories of practice, approaches to intervening in these problems highlight the porosity of boundaries and bodies and their emergent materialities as they continuously intermingle in practices across time and space, redefining notions of risk, responsibility and control.

4

CONCEPTUALISING MICROBIAL MATERIALITY BEYOND SIMPLE CATEGORIES

Cecily Maller

Introduction

Microbes are microscopic organisms of many different kinds found almost everywhere on earth (Yong, 2016). There are an estimated trillion microbial species (Rappuoli et al., 2023) varying across different environments and practices (Maller, 2023). They occur as populations of single species, in communities and as complex microbiomes. The main types include bacteria, fungi, viruses and single-celled creatures such as protozoa. First seen under microscopes in the 17th Century by English and Dutch scientists Robert Hooke and Antoni van Leeuwenhoek (Gest, 2004), microbes are otherwise more or less invisible to the naked human eye, highly mobile and in constant exchange inside and outside bodies, traversing most environmental boundaries (Robinson et al., 2020). People could inhale up to one hundred million microbes each day (Després et al., 2012). In indoor settings, people also contribute substantially to microbiomes via constant exchanges of breath, touch, and other forms of 'shedding' (Meadow et al., 2015). With such constant exchanges, human and other bodies are ensconced in microbial flows.

After being neglected in recent decades by scientists and social theorists alike, in the last 10 years microbes have 'migrated from the ... fringes of biology to its spotlight-hogging centre' (Yong, 2016: 249). Supported by increasingly fine-tuned technologies able to detect microbial species and their traces, considerable knowledge is being developed that reveals details about the materiality, functionality and relationality of microbes and microbiomes in a range of environments, bodies and ecologies (e.g., Wakefield-Rann, 2021). The threat of pandemics, the rise of AMR, and the generation of new

DOI: 10.4324/9781003685210-6

knowledge about the human health benefits of contact with microbiomes, have turned the spotlight on human-microbial relations. A classic case is the COVID-19 pandemic which changed practices of health, hygiene, working, travelling and socialising on a global scale associated with scientific, technological and policy responses (Caroppo et al., 2021). This and other examples serve as a stark reminder that microbes are always inextricably part of social worlds. But despite elevated fears post-COVID-19, only a very small number of human-microbial relations are generally harmful (Yong, 2016). The majority are fundamental for health and immunity (Robinson and Breed, 2023).

Based on a deliberately post-Pasteurian view (Paxson, 2008), this chapter works through some of the ways that human-microbial relations and microbial materiality are conceptualised in social practice theory. Although grounded in literature on theories of social practice, the chapter also draws on a wide range of recent research about microbes and human-microbial relations from other disciplines including microbiology, health and geography that highlight their complex relationality. Social practice theory is not introduced here except to explain that social practices comprise material arrangements, or combinations of different materials, meanings and skills (Shove et al., 2012; Schatzki, 2010), are perpetuated over time and space through regular 'performances' (Reckwitz, 2002), and are connected with other practices to form larger complexes and networks (Hui et al., 2017). Their materiality varies widely depending on the type of activity and where, when and how it takes place, as is amply illustrated by the broad literature on social practices (e.g., Kuijer, 2019; Nicolini, 2012; Rinkinen et al., 2019).

Materials that take the form of resources and their infrastructures have been a particular feature of practice theory research (Wilhite, 2008; Cahill et al., 2024). A classic example is a subset of work on energy and water demand in everyday life. In this literature, materials have a dual conceptualisation in that they are viewed both as infrastructures that enable certain practices to be carried out as well as being resources that practices consume. Heating and cooling homes or offices (Hitchings, 2011), washing clothes, bodies, and dishes (Kuijer, 2019), and other practices that use energy or water feature strongly (Strengers et al., 2022; Kadibadiba et al., 2018). The artefacts accounted for in these practices such as taps, appliances and switches denote the presence of energy and water, but the materiality of the resources themselves is rarely discussed. One reason may be that because the research problems studied have focused on consumption and sustainability it makes sense to focus on the appliances and technologies that 'deliver' resources in a useable form. Similar articles studying food consumption (Middha and Lewis, 2021) also highlight the typical materialities most literature on social practices has described: tangible, (often) discrete and consumable (Maller and Strengers, 2019).

Expanding ways of thinking about materiality has led to exploration of how more varied 'materials', including human and non-human bodies, might be represented in and understood through social practices (Blue, 2025). For example, Maller (2025) discusses the ongoing co-constitution between bodies and practices, describing how bodies contribute materially to practices while practices simultaneously leave imprints on bodies. The changes practices inscribe on bodies in turn affect material and mental capacities through epigenetic and other mechanisms. Blue (2025) goes further in that his processual account of the dynamics of practices overtly collapses the subject-object divide and the distinctions between practices and those who do them. He makes several theoretical moves to consider the doers of practices as 'dividual' which means bodies are part of shared social assemblages, the medium and site of practice connections, and are constantly in a state of emergence (Blue, 2025). Although they take very different approaches to the topic, Blue and Maller suppose that bodies and by extension, materials, are multiple, unbounded and always ongoing, in contrast to the singular, bounded and static status assigned to them by most contemporary Western thought (Shove et al., 2024).

Delving further into other ways of thinking about materiality suggests that a multitude of microbes are involved in very mundane, but very necessary, functions and roles in human and other bodies, and that they make sure things hum along through time and space. Having accepted the idea of bodies being multiple, how could social practice theory contribute to further understanding human-microbial relations and help reframe pervasive antimicrobial narratives?

The first section of this chapter explores how the materialities of microbes and microbial communities are included in the theorisation and analysis of social practices. It describes how conceptualising human-microbial relations through social practices resolves oft-cited binaries, which have been critiqued in other literature (Beck, 2021; Hird, 2010). It also explains how social practice accounts avoid the trap of categorising microbes as one type of material or another, or having one type of material effect. Building on these ideas, the second section turns to what this means for complex questions about how to respond to challenges arising from human-microbial relations, including pandemics and the problem of AMR, and starts to reframe everyday relations with microbes and microbiomes in various settings. The conclusion reviews the implications of these arguments and asks what considerations of microbial materiality mean for social practice theory.

Microbial materiality in social practices

In conceptualising microbial materiality using social practice theory, perhaps the most obvious place to start is to contemplate microbes and microbial communities as part of the materiality or material arrangements of practices (Shove et al., 2026). In the context of the discussion so far presented in this chapter, microbes are abundantly part of human or other bodies involved in carrying out practices and they create effects through their presence or absence in both bodies and environments (e.g., in gut health, disease). Microbes are also components of the materials or resources consumed by practices, particularly food – where they also have an undeniable role in much of its production (e.g., cheese, wine, bread, beer) (Paxson, 2008) – but also in water, air and other elements.

Distinct characteristics of microbes that for some may challenge their conceptualisation as material arrangements include their capacity to very rapidly adapt and evolve in response to stimuli or changed conditions and, more importantly, their specific roles in particular practices. Examples include their recruitment into new practices to solve environmental and health problems, such as reducing plastic waste (Carpenter, 2021), making energy (Carrington, 2021), and curing cancer (Shepherd, 2022). Other practices involved in the treatment of disease also rely on the specific ecologies and functions of microbes. Examples include faecal microbiota transplantation (Shepherd, 2022) and the use of bacteriophages to treat antimicrobial infections (Kuchment, 2012). With these developments, could microbes be considered more than part of material arrangements and instead potentially also be a type of performer of practice alongside and with humans?

In some types of practice theory research around the 2010s, people are considered to be the main performers and carriers of practices (Gram-Hanssen, 2009). But thinking around this idea is not consistent as a variety of non-humans and materials and their various constitution in and by practices have been considered (Gherardi, 2025; Maller and Strengers, 2019,;Schatzki, 2010), in tandem with broader scholarly discussions of post-humanism that challenge human-centrism (Castree and Nash, 2006; Braidotti, 2018). The practice theory literature includes the specific theorisation of non-human species as well as inanimate and animate objects as part of practices. Some authors go as far to suggest that non-human species could also carry out practices and share skills and meanings, including pets and plants (Strengers et al., 2016; Hitchings, 2003). However, despite the temptation to elevate non-human agencies and capacities, particularly in practices where microbes or other species have distinct or essential roles, in a true practice ontology, agency and performance lies with practices themselves and their formation in patterns of bundles and complexes. In other words, agency is not attributed to one or more components, either performers or materials (Shove et al., 2012; Blue, 2025). By way of explaining further, Shove et al. (2024; 2026) conceptualise social practices as sites of biosocial becoming, collapsing distinctions between biological and social materialities and activities. These authors explain how 'related practices, and combinations of them, generate distinctive and spatially uneven interactions between microbes and other organisms, including humans' (Shove et al., 2024: 166). Taking an inclusive and fluid view of materiality and performativity makes it possible to describe the myriad ways that microbes, biological processes and events (Schatzki, 2019; Meloni, 2018) are part of, enable, interrupt, prompt and intersect in all practices.

Approaches that firmly ascribe agency to one or more actors or components of practices, or that engage in detailed discussions about particular material or other capabilities, lean towards individualistic or siloed ways of thinking rather than consistently adopting a social practice ontology (Hui et al., 2017). In other words, in these scenarios, people, microbes, or some other entity quickly become the conceptual and analytical starting point rather than starting with practices (Shove et al., 2024; Hui et al., 2017). More practically, conceptualising microbes in one discrete category or another (i.e., material, material effect, or performer) limits what social practice theory can offer in addressing current human-microbial challenges. With their omnipresence, complex communities and shapeshifting abilities in different places and times, microbes resist fixed classification. This understanding can be transferred to other material streams that flow through practices which also don't have the sharp edges of objects or things or the programmable features of technologies and software; materials that similarly resist straightforward classification in social theories, including chemical, physical and biological processes and their compositions (Schatzki, 2019; Blue, 2025), allergens, or other micro or nano particles (Wakefield-Rann, 2021; Meloni and Maller, 2024).

What is evident from this discussion and increasingly argued in social practice and other related theoretical scholarship (Blue, 2025; Meloni, 2018; Shove et al., 2024), is that practices always involve complex flows of biosocial matter, much more than any obvious, observable materialities or subjectivities. In the case of epidemics and pandemics, many, if not most of practices of everyday life can be reshaped, paused or irrevocably changed seemingly by the activities of a single microbial species, according to conventional views. But a social practices ontology sees the problem differently. It understands any observable disease outcome to be the manifestation of historical complexes and networks of practices of various kinds that have shaped human-microbial relations in particular directions, whether intended or otherwise. This feature of social practices enables conversations about change and momentum to consider dynamics across space and time compared to behavioural or other approaches that narrowly focus on the agencies or attitudes, behaviours and choices of people (Shove, 2010) or the doings of things or other species, microbe or not, in any given moment.

Moving beyond antimicrobial narratives to understand human-microbial relations through social practices

Although there has been a recent probiotic shift (Lorimer, 2020; Greenhough et al., 2018), most social research on microbes has concentrated on the harmful effects of disease (Hinchliffe, 2022; Lupton, 2022). However, as Lorimer (2017: 533) explains, 'no microbe is essentially pathogenic; pathogenesis is the outcome of political and ecological relations'. In fact, traditional scientific research is showing that too few microbes in both environments and bodies are associated with multiple chronic inflammatory diseases and conditions caused by poorly functioning immunity, including Alzheimer's (Sochocka et al., 2019), asthma, allergies, bowel and skin diseases, obesity, and depression (Robinson et al., 2020; Lorimer, 2017). New evidence from microbiology demonstrates that long-term exposure to diverse microbiomes over the life course protects against inflammation and chronic disease conditions, including asthma and dementia (Robinson et al., 2020; Flies et al., 2017), contrasting with previous Pasteurian ways of managing microbes that focused on elimination (Paxson, 2008). This knowledge is prompting various developments in practice and policy and represents an opportunity for more widespread change. For example, building codes are being reviewed in Asia because of new insights into how design and management practices can support 'healthy' exposure to microbes through the use of construction materials, the function and use of spaces, and changes in sunlight, ventilation, humidity, temperature and other variables (Villoria et al., 2025). Given that people typically spend up to 90% of their time indoors (Morawska et al., 2024), understanding how practices can change indoor airborne microbiomes (aerobiomes) and contact with other microbiomes and vice versa will be a critical area of exploration for understanding and improving human health and immunity.

Meanwhile, in high-income countries, antimicrobial sentiments and narratives of hypercleanliness have become entrenched in family, work and healthcare settings (Wakefield-Rann, 2021), giving rise to new technologies and products and changing the trajectories of existing practices. For example, there is increased anxiety about air and airborne microbes, particularly shared air in indoor spaces (Lupton, 2022; Strengers et al., 2024) prompting proliferation of carbon dioxide monitors, sterilisation technologies and air filters to ostensibly remove 99% of microbes from buildings and rooms (Meloni and Maller, 2024). Although practices in healthcare settings and institutions are highly regulated, microbial management in everyday life is not and it is where disinfectants, chemicals and cleanliness practices (and the marketing of them) can result in the over- or under-sterilisation of bodies, buildings, and indoor environments (Wakefield-Rann, 2021). Regarding antibiotic use, over prescription and incomplete administration are the most dangerous. Resistant microbes and their genes spread through environmental microbiomes (Hashmi, 2020), albeit unevenly (Hinchliffe, 2022), and there is an increase in the number of antimicrobial resistant infections in people, pets, and agricultural animals (Landecker, 2016). The implications of global AMR for humans and other species are vastly underappreciated in terms of the threat this represents to one of the most effective treatments for disease (antibiotics) and the potential it has to 'undo' many of the gains of modern medicine and agriculture, including the elimination of devastating diseases in human populations and the ability to intensively produce livestock and crops.

As these examples show, in general, approaches to manage human-microbial interactions are reactive, blunt and clumsy, equivalent to a scorched earth policy. Products and practices often attempt to essentially annihilate all microbiota in any given environment, rather than only targeting those that are problematic in that setting or adopting other measures that might involve rebalancing microbial communities or understanding and managing infection and contamination in other ways, as many chapters in this volume illustrate. A large part of the problem in many scenarios is the method of treating all microbes with equivalence (as foes) and the use of nonspecific antimicrobial products and technologies. What is urgently needed is a move away from simple binaries of 'good' and 'bad' or 'friend' or 'foe' (as applied to microbes, environments, people, and other animals who may be potential vectors) to consider the biosocial dimensions of a wide range of practices that collectively result in emergence, distribution and patterning of human-microbial relations (Shove et al., 2024). In addition, narratives and meanings of human-microbial relations need to be reframed from being overwhelmingly negative to more affirmative, adaptive and probiotic heading towards what could be described as a form of post-Pasteurian stewardship.

There are several ways social practice theory could support the development of more probiotic human-microbial relations. The first is to start with social practice theory as a conceptual framework to develop a detailed understanding of the roles of different material arrangements, skills and meanings in shaping historical and contemporary practices that directly respond to and impact microbial communities in both every day and professional settings. The second would include mapping and linking complexes of practices and their constituent elements across various sectors, industries, geographies and communities, to understand how they collectively impact microbiomes and exposures to them, and how they may be contributing to or tackling antibiosis, hypercleanliness and other problems. In following the microbial or biotic impacts from linking these practices as complex networks, the collective and specific impacts on microbiomes could be monitored in ways that complement existing strategies. In revealing where there are unexpected co-dependent connections across practices that may not have been revealed before, new strategies to intervene could be developed. Although it may be controversial, and although it might not be possible to control change in this way, a third option is to encourage and develop new 'microbially responsible' practices through policy, regulation and the adjustment of standards. For example, new practices of designing buildings with probiotic materials, implementing ventilation technologies and changing how they are used in air management could support exposure to the sorts of microbiomes human health is either dependent upon or benefits from. The role of microbes in achieving or thwarting desired public health outcomes through social practices could be recognised, valued and shared, enriching the meanings and teleology of practices without treating microbes or people or something else as either 'the problem' or 'the solution'.

The practices of everyday life, including hygiene, cleanliness, comfort and consumption, appear to offer an obvious starting point. However, focusing only on domestic settings and excluding professional ones would fail to achieve the comprehensive approach that is needed. Social practice theory could be used to develop a common language to facilitate dialogue across disciplines and across professional and domestic environments, particularly where there is contrasting, conflicting or impartial knowledge about microbes and microbiomes. Dialogue supported by shared meanings, knowing and doings could be used to guide the development of technologies, policies and practices to be implemented in ways that are deliberately protective against under- or over-exposure to microbes, or exposure to particular ones known to be harmful in certain scenarios. For example, interventions or approaches grounded in social practices could reinvigorate policy-making and building codes in healthcare and educational settings where people spend significant time and are constantly exposed to indoor air, such as schools, universities, hospitals and care facilities for the elderly. Accompanying these policies and codes, new narratives of stewardship and meanings about microbial care could be introduced into practices of hygiene and commensality to move beyond overly simplified binaries of 'good' and 'bad' germs. In some social circles affirmative microbial narratives are already present, for example in probiotic health and organic food movements (Lorimer, 2017), and in clinical settings where antimicrobial resistant infections have led to probiotic alternatives, such as phage therapy (Gordillo Altamirano and Barr, 2019). In these ways, social practice theories could support a move toward microbial stewardship that encompasses the diverse and changing microbiomes that characterise human-microbial and other more-than-human relations.

As understanding about microbial ecologies is extended, deepened and shared, narratives about human-microbial relations could 'naturally' shift towards the affirmative. However, it is not likely to be enough to counter entrenched meanings of antimicrobiality and the practices it is part of or be sufficient to resolve increasing occurrences of AMR. Whatever the approach, multisectoral, cooperative, long-term strategies will be required.

Conclusion

The main task for this chapter has been to show how microbial materiality is conceptualised using a social practice ontology and how such framings help to understand the intricacies of human-microbial relations in ways that account for complexity and nuance. It has explored how microbes and microbial ecologies are reproduced, taking into consideration the possibility that they could be seen as types of materials and performers of practice, and then settling on a position that represents them as part of biosocial flows through and comprising practices. Although there may be no single 'right' way to conceptualise microbes in social practices, there is strong appeal in adopting an approach that accounts for multiple processes and material flows that enable the dissolution of boundaries between practices, bodies and environments. To reiterate, the specific theorisation will always be dependent on the relevant human-microbial relations at play, the practices of empirical concern and the questions that need answers in any given place and time. However, conceptualising human-microbial relations using theories of social practice is consistent with other literature that moves beyond simple binaries while also illustrating how microbes resist simplistic material classifications.

The chapter then turned to what a social practice theoretical conceptualisation means for understanding complex questions regarding human-microbial relations, including responding to pandemics, tackling the problem of AMR, and starting to reframe everyday relations with microbes and microbiomes in various scenarios and settings. With headlines that are usually based on biased and negative storylines, focusing on social practices is one way human-microbial relations in advanced urban economies can be reframed from a state of anxiety post-COVID-19 towards post-Pasteurian notions of stewardship.

Finally, it might be worth reflecting on what trying to conceptualise the materiality of microbes within practices brings to social practice theory. At a basic level, it shows that practices always involve multiple bodies, human and non-human. It also highlights the fluidity of edges and boundaries, the constant biosocial connections between practices, and the complexities of biological and other processes, most of which are rarely observable. These developments help push the theory further away from a human-centric focus on practitioners or performers and might also be relevant to understanding other complex biosocial relations, including between other human and non-human species, and other micro-entities such as genes, and chemicals. As new scientific knowledge and techniques enable greater understanding of the lives of microbes and microbiomes and their impacts and contributions, further questions will arise about how, why and when such entities matter for practice-based accounts of the world and vice versa.

References

Beck, A. (2021). 'Microbiomes as companion species: an exploration of dis- and re-entanglements with the microbial self', *Social and Cultural Geography,* 22: 357–375. https://doi.org/10.1080/14649365.2019.1593490.

Blue, S. (2025). *Practice Theory and Process Philosophy: Towards a sociology of becoming*. London: Routledge. https://doi.org/10.4324/9781032685175.

Braidotti, R. (2018). 'A Theoretical Framework for the Critical Posthumanities', *Theory, Culture and Society,* 36: 31–61. https://doi.org/10.1177/0263276418771486.

Cahill, J., Hoolohan, C. and Browne, A. (2024). 'Social practice theory and household water demand: A review of literature and research evidence', *WIREs Water,* 11: e1719. https://doi.org/10.1002/wat2.1719.

Caroppo, E., Mazza, M., Sannella, A., Marano, G., Avallone, C., Claro, A. E., Janiri, D., Moccia, L., Janiri, L. and Sani, G. (2021). 'Will Nothing Be the Same Again?: Changes in Lifestyle during COVID-19 Pandemic and Consequences on Mental Health', *International journal of environmental research and public health,* 18: 8433. https://doi.org/10.3390/ijerph18168433.

Carpenter, S. (2021). 'The Race To Develop Plastic-Eating Bacteria', *Forbes*, 10/3/2021.

Carrington, D. (2021). 'Microbes and solar power "could produce 10 times more food than plants"', *The Guardian*, 22/06/2021.

Castree, N. and Nash, C. (2006). 'Posthuman geographies', *Social and Cultural Geography,* 7: 501–504. https://doi.org/10.1080/14649360600825620.

Després, V., Huffman, J., Burrows, S., Hoose, C., Safatov, A., Buryak, G., Fröhlich-Nowoisky, J., Elbert, W., Andreae, M., Pöschl, U., and Jaenicke, R. (2012). 'Primary biological aerosol particles in the atmosphere: a review', *Tellus B: Chemical and Physical Meteorology*, *64*(1). doi.org/10.3402/tellusb.v64i0.15598 works for me.

Flies, E. J., Skelly, C., Negi, S. S., Prabhakaran, P., Liu, Q., Liu, K., Goldizen, F. C., Lease, C. and Weinstein, P. (2017). 'Biodiverse green spaces: a prescription for global urban health', *Frontiers in Ecology and the Environment,* 15: 510–516. https://doi.org/10.1002/fee.1630.

Gest, H. (2004). 'The discovery of microorganisms by Robert Hooke and Antoni van Leeuwenhoek, Fellows of The Royal Society', *Notes and Records of the Royal Society of London,* 58: 187–201. https://doi.org/10.1098/rsnr.2004.0055.

Gherardi, S. (2025). 'What is the Place of the Human Being in Practice Theories? An Answer from a Posthumanist Position', *The Journal of Practice Theory,* 1. https://doi.org/10.71936/wkm2-9s32.

Gordillo Altamirano, F. L. and Barr, J. J. (2019). 'Phage Therapy in the Postantibiotic Era', *Clinical microbiology reviews*, 32. https://doi.org/10.1128/cmr.00066-18.

Gram-Hanssen, K. (2009). 'Standby consumption in households analyzed with a practice theory approach', *Journal of Industrial Ecology,* 14: 150–165. https://doi.org/10.1111/j.1530-9290.2009.00194.x.

Greenhough, B., Dwyer, A., Grenyer, R., Hodgetts, T., McLeod, C. and Lorimer, J. (2018). 'Unsettling antibiosis: how might interdisciplinary researchers generate a feeling for the microbiome and to what effect?', *Palgrave Communications,* 4: 149. https://doi.org/10.1057/s41599-018-0196-3.

Hashmi, M. Z. (2020). *Antibiotics and Antimicrobial Resistance Genes in the Environment*. Amsterdam, Netherlands: Elsevier. eBook ISBN: 9780128188835.

Hinchliffe, S. (2022). 'Postcolonial Global Health, Post-Colony Microbes and Antimicrobial Resistance', *Theory, Culture and Society,* 39: 145–168. https://doi.org/10.1177/0263276420981606.

Hird, M. J. (2010). 'Meeting with the Microcosmos', *Environment and Planning D: Society and Space,* 28: 36–39. https://doi.org/10.1068/d2706wsc.

Hitchings, R. (2003). 'People, plants and performance: on actor network theory and the material pleasures of the private garden', *Social and Cultural Geography,* 4: 99–114. https://doi.org/10.1080/1464936032000049333.

Hitchings, R. (2011). 'Researching air-conditioning addiction and ways of puncturing practice: professional office workers and the decision to go outside', *Environment and Planning A,* 43: 2838–2856. https://doi.org/10.1068/a43574.

Hui, A., Schatzki, T. and Shove, E. (eds) (2017). *The Nexus of Practices: Connections, constellations, practitioners.* London: Routledge. https://doi.org/10.4324/9781315560816.

Kadibadiba, T., Roberts, L. and Duncan, R. (2018). 'Living in a city without water: A social practice theory analysis of resource disruption in Gaborone, Botswana', *Global Environmental Change,* 53: 273–285. https://doi.org/10.1016/j.gloenvcha.2018.10.005.

Kuchment, A. (2012). *The Forgotten Cure: The past and future of phage therapy,* New York: Springer. https://doi.org/10.1007/978-1-4614-0251-0.

Kuijer, L. (2019). 'Automated Artefacts as Co-performers of Social Practices: Washing Machines, Laundering and Design' in Maller, C. and Strengers, Y. (eds.) *Social Practices and Dynamic Non-Humans: Nature, Materials and Technologies.* London: Palgrave Macmillan. https://doi.org/10.1007/978-3-319-92189-1_10.

Landecker, H. (2016). 'Antibiotic Resistance and the Biology of History', *Body and Society,* 22: 19–52. https://doi.org/10.1177/1357034X14561341.

Lorimer, J. (2017). 'Parasites, ghosts and mutualists: a relational geography of microbes for global health', *Transactions of the Institute of British Geographers,* 42: 544–558. http://www.jstor.org/stable/45147116.

Lorimer, J. (2020). *The Probiotic Planet: Using life to manage life.* Minneapolis: University of Minnesota Press. https://doi.org/10.5749/j.ctv19cw9vg.

Lupton, D. (2022). *COVID Societies: Theorising the Coronavirus crisis.* Oxford: Routledge. https://doi.org/10.4324/9781003200512.

Maller, C. (2023). 'Resetting urban human-microbial relations in pandemic times'. *Geography compass,* 17: e12680. https://doi.org/10.1111/gec3.12680.

Maller, C. (2025). 'Proposing a Gradient of Humanism/Non-Humanism and Understanding The Contributions of Body-Minds To Social Practices'. *The Journal of Practice Theory*, 1. https://doi.org/10.71936/58z1-2h89.

Maller, C. and Strengers, Y. (eds.) (2019). *Social practices and dynamic non-humans: Nature, materials and technologies.* London: Palgrave Macmillan. https://doi.org/10.1007/978-3-319-92189-1.

Meadow, J. F., Altrichter, A. E., Bateman, A. C., Stenson, J., Brown, G. Z., Green, J. L. and Bohannan, B. J. M. (2015). 'Humans differ in their personal microbial cloud', *PeerJ,* San Francisco, CA. 3: e1258–e1258. https://doi.org/10.7717/peerj.1258.

Meloni, M. (2018). 'A Postgenomic Body: Histories, Genealogy, Politics', *Body and Society,* 24: 3–38. https://doi.org/10.1177/1357034X18785445.

Meloni, M. and Maller, C. (2024). 'Revitalizing Air: More-than-Human Relations in Urban Health Beyond the Modern-Premodern Binary', *GeoHumanities,* 10: 56–72. https://doi.org/10.1080/2373566X.2023.2280570.

Middha, B. and Lewis, T. (2021). 'Pop-up food provisioning as a sustainable third space: reshaping eating practices at an inner urban university', *Australian geographer,* 52: 407–424. https://doi.org/10.1080/00049182.2021.2017250.

Morawska, L., Allen, J., Bahnfleth, W., Bennett, B., Bluyssen, P. M., Boerstra, A., Buonanno, G., Cao, J., Dancer, S. J., Floto, A., Franchimon, F., Greenhalgh, T., Haworth, C., Hogeling, J., Isaxon, C., Jimenez, J. L., Kennedy, A., Kumar, P., Kurnitski, J., Li, Y., Loomans, M., Marks, G., Marr, L. C., Mazzarella, L., Melikov, A. K., Miller, S. L., Milton, D. K., Monty, J., Nielsen, P. V., Noakes, C., Peccia, J., Prather, K. A., Querol, X., Salthammer, T., Sekhar, C., Seppänen, O., Tanabe, S.-I., Tang, J. W., Tellier, R., Tham, K. W., Wargocki, P., Wierzbicka, A. and Yao, M. (2024). 'Mandating indoor air quality for public buildings', *Science,* 383: 1418–1420. https://doi.org/10.1126/science.adl0677.

Nicolini, D. (2012). *Practice Theory, Work, and Organization: An introduction.* Oxford: Oxford University Press. e ISBN: 9780191644627

Paxson, H. (2008). 'Post-Pasteurian Cultures: The microbiopolitics of raw-milk cheese in the United States', *Cultural Anthropology,* 23: 15–47. https://doi.org/10.1111/j.1548-1360.2008.00002.x.

Rappuoli, R., Young, P., Ron, E., Pecetta, S. and Pizza, M. (2023). 'Save the microbes to save the planet. A call to action of the International Union of the Microbiological Societies (IUMS)', *One Health Outlook,* 5: 5. https://doi.org/10.1186/s42522-023-00077-2.

Reckwitz, A. (2002). 'Toward a Theory of Social Practices: A Development in Culturalist Theorizing', *European Journal of Social Theory,* 5: 243–263. https://doi.org/10.1177/13684310222225432.

Rinkinen, J., Shove, E. and Smits, M. (2019). 'Cold chains in Hanoi and Bangkok: Changing systems of provision and practice', *Journal of Consumer Culture,* 19: 379–397. https://doi.org/10.1177/1469540517717783.

Robinson, J. M. and Breed, M. F. (2023). 'The aerobiome–health axis: a paradigm shift in bioaerosol thinking', *Trends in Microbiology,* 3: 661–664. https://doi.org/10.1016/j.tim.2023.04.007.

Robinson, J. M., Cando-Dumancela, C., Liddicoat, C., Weinstein, P., Cameron, R. and Breed, M. F. (2020). 'Vertical Stratification in Urban Green Space Aerobiomes', *Environmental health perspectives,* 128: 117008. https://pmc.ncbi.nlm.nih.gov/articles/PMC7687659/.

Schatzki, T. (2010). 'Materiality and Social Life', *Nature and Culture,* 5: 123–149. https://doi.org/10.3167/nc.2010.050202.

Schatzki, T. (2019). *Social Change in a Material World: How activity and material processes dynamize practices.* London: Routledge. https://doi.org/10.4324/9780429032127.

Shepherd, T. (2022). 'Super poo: the emerging science of stool transplants and designer gut bacteria', *The Guardian,* 3/1/2022.

Shove, E. (2010). 'Beyond the ABC: Climate Change Policy and Theories of Social Change', *Environment and Planning A,* 42: 1273–1285. https://doi.org/10.1068/a42282.

Shove, E., Blue, S. and Kelly, M. P. (2024). 'Categorising and cohabiting: practices as the site of biosocial becoming', *Social Theory and Health,* 22: 156–171. https://doi.org/10.1057/s41285-024-00204-7.

Shove, E., Blue, S. and Kelly, M. P. (2026). *Practice Theory and the Biosocial: Microbes, matter and milieu.* Oxford: Berghahn. https://doi.org/10.3167/9781836953395.

Shove, E., Pantzar, M. and Watson, M. (2012). *The Dynamics of Social Practice: Everyday life and how it changes*. London: Sage. https://doi.org/10.4135/9781446250655.

Sochocka, M., Donskow-Łysoniewska, K., Diniz, B. S., Kurpas, D., Brzozowska, E. and Leszek, J. (2019). 'The Gut Microbiome Alterations and Inflammation-Driven Pathogenesis of Alzheimer's Disease—a Critical Review', *Molecular neurobiology*, 56: 1841–1851. https://doi.org/10.1007/s12035-018-1188-4.

Strengers, Y., Gram-Hanssen, K., Dahlgren, K. and Aagaard, L. K. (2022). 'Energy, emerging technologies and gender in homes', *Buildings and Cities*, 3: 842–853. https://doi.org/10.5334/bc.273.

Strengers, Y., Nicholls, L. and Maller, C. (2016). 'Curious energy consumers: Humans and non-humans in assemblages of household practice', *Journal of Consumer Culture*, 16: 761–780. https://doi.org/10.1177/1469540514536194.

Strengers, Y., Pink, S., Dahlgren, K. and Korsmeyer, H. (2024). 'Healthy, safe and comfortable: Emerging indoor air practices in Australian households', *Energy Research and Social Science*, 118: 103760. https://doi.org/10.1016/j.erss.2024.103760.

Villoria, M. B. D., Argayosa, V. B., Rosalinas, A. D., Valerio, D. N. R., La Madrid, C. L. and Ticzon, M. X. N. (2025). 'Integrating building code to microbial count studies in urban built spaces with ventilation and human presence: a model', *Frontiers in built environment*, 10. https://doi.org/10.3389/fbuil.2024.1517638.

Wakefield-Rann, R. (2021). *Life Indoors: How our homes are shaping our bodies and our planet*. Singapore: Springer Link. https://doi.org/10.1007/978-981-16-5176-2.

Wilhite, H. (2008). 'New thinking on the agentive relationship between end-use technologies and energy-using practices', *Energy Efficiency*, 1: 121–130. https://doi.org/10.1007/s12053-008-9006-x.

Yong, E. (2016). *I Contain Multitudes: The miicrobes within us and a grander view of life*. London: The Bodley Head. https://doi.org/10.22339/jbh.v1i1.2245.

5

MICROBIOME REPAIR

Probiotic practices in agriculture

George Cusworth, Beth Greenhough and Jamie Lorimer

Introduction

Recent reports have highlighted the environmental costs of modern agricultural systems in terms of their impact on soil and on human and animal health (Montgomery et al., 2024). Viewed through a microbial lens, these changes can be understood as a breakdown of the relationship between humans and microbes arising from changes in agricultural practice. The 'treadmill' (Van Den Bosch, 1978) of intensive tillage, which sees soil frequently disturbed through practices such as ploughing and harrowing, and the use of agrochemicals such as fertilisers, herbicides and pesticides, strips soils, crops and livestock of the microbial diversity needed to sustain fertility and resist disease (Singh et al., 2020). This increased vulnerability is then addressed through the further use of agrochemical inputs, such as antibiotics, creating a negative feedback cycle of dependence, damage and disease. Collectively we refer to this program of agricultural intensification, characterised by large-scale monocultures, a reliance on chemical inputs and a focus on high yields (Hartmann and Six, 2023) as the antibiotic model (Lorimer, 2020).

The antibiotic approach to agriculture has been linked to the dramatic rise in antimicrobial resistance or AMR, with implications for both human and animal health (Woolhouse et al., 2015) and to reductions in the ability of the soil microbiome to deliver environmental goods such as the sequestration of carbon, the regulation of the water cycle, and the production of nutrient-rich food (Nasem, 2024). These are some of the risks (Beck, 1992), blowbacks (Wallace and Wallace, 2015) or unintended consequences of past rounds of agricultural modernisation and associated dysbiosis (Frąc et al., 2022). These

DOI: 10.4324/9781003685210-7

moments, when agricultural systems break down, simultaneously open up a space where social science analyses can draw attention to the necessity of ongoing care, maintenance and repair (Puig de la Bellacasa, 2015).

One response to these shifts within social science has been to draw attention to how the risks of microbial dysbiosis or blowback are governed. For example, in her analysis of the human-microbial relations associated with raw milk cheese making in Vermont, Paxson (2008) develops the concept of microbiopolitics to describe how knowledge about microbes is deployed to govern human and non-human life. This maintains the Pasteurian focus on minimising the circulation of pathogenic microbes while seeking to ensure the preservation and circulation of beneficial microbes and human-microbial interactions. Paxson is emblematic of a growing number of social scientists examining the science of the microbiome and a wider 'microbiomania' (Paxson and Helmreich, 2014) associated with the popularisation of knowledge of the microbiome, which has given rise to probiotic modes of microbiopolitics in healthcare (Lorimer, 2020; Beck, 2021), waste management (Zhang, 2024) and food production (Cusworth and Lorimer, 2024).

In this chapter we also take the need for microbial repair as our starting point but turn to focus on the biosocial farming practices through which probiotic modes of governance are enacted. Microbial repair, as we have defined elsewhere, involves

> [r]eversing the damage done by an intensive model of agricultural management predicated on agroecological simplification and high inputs of fertilizers, pesticides, and antibiotics. This is achieved through the cultivation of functional and resilient microbial ecologies capable of reversing the blowbacks caused by microbial dysbiosis. It demands careful attention to how microbes interact with one another, and with other biotic and abiotic factors to deliver key agricultural functions. It seeks a just and sustainable food system that is healthy for people and the planet.
>
> *(Cusworth et al., 2025: 1)*

Post-Pasteurian microbiome repair aims to secure or restore a desired system state: to fix the dysbiosis seen as the root cause of many of the blowbacks outlined above. Where a Pasteurian approach focused on isolating and eliminating pathogenic microbes, a post-Pasteurian approach positions at least some microbes as active collaborators who work with humans to coproduce healthy soils, crops and livestock. Working with microbes is seen as a way of intervening in shared metabolic processes, such as digestion (within livestock bodies) and decomposition, to deliver more sustainable, healthy and balanced agricultural systems. Repair is enabled through the strategic deployment of (or collaboration with) individual organisms. This might involve the 'symbiotic engineering' of livestock through, for example, changing patterns of tilling and grazing to allow fungi and bacteria to build soil carbon (Cusworth et al., 2022), or adding legumes to crop rotations to enable soil bacteria to fix nitrogen thereby modulating biogeochemical interactions at the earth-life interface. Table 5.1 lists different kinds of probiotic practices, all of which seek to intervene in human-microbe relations on the farm.

This approach situates farming practices previously understood as human-directed and controlled – such as fertilisation and cultivation – as biosocial practices (Shove et al., 2024): as much the product of non-human microbial agency as of human action or chemical processes. Similarly, soils once seen as inert substrates or infrastructure, are now being reimagined within farming systems as co-produced through human and non-human practices, reflected in agronomy through a move towards concepts of *soil health* and away from terms like *soil fertility* or *soil quality* (Lehmann et al., 2020). Krzywoszynska (2019) describes how this new ontology for agriculture can involve abandoning, or at least minimising, long-established farming practices such as tilling the soil, and developing new skills in soil care focused on improving soil structure and composition. Significantly, these practices are not those humans can carry out in isolation.

In the analysis that follows we identify three bundles (after Schatzki, 2002) of biosocial farming practices orientated towards microbial repair that we term attunement, co-cultivation and collective care, paying attention to the meanings (understandings and rationales), materials (technologies and infrastructures) and competencies (skills and practical know-how) involved in each (after Shove et al., 2012). This argument is illustrated with reference to a range of examples drawn from ongoing research into the microbiopolitics of agricultural production in the UK. The observations we discuss have emerged from ethnographic and interview-based encounters with regenerative agriculturalists, agronomists, crop and soil scientists, commercial arable farmers, food system policymakers, conservation charities and farming advocacy groups and agricultural union bodies. To help narrate these empirical engagements, we also draw on social and natural science writing on the agronomic, cultural and economic aspects of managing agroecosystems and the microbial configurations that co-constitute them.

We then consider what paying attention to biosocial farming practices reveals about different forms of microbial repair, their antecedents and their capacities for transformation. We trace the practical means through which microbial relations are reconfigured to secure desired relations, demonstrating how nexuses of biosocial practices interconnect to act at scale (Hui et al., 2016), and we draw on the distinction between repair-as-maintenance and repair-as-transformation (Henke and Sims, 2020) to note that meaningful repair may need to challenge and transform status quo approaches to deliver soil, human and animal health.

TABLE 5.1 Illustrative examples of agricultural microbial repair

	Farm type	*Practice*	*Purposes*	*Repair through*
Supplementary practices	Broiler chickens	Microbes – specifically *Lactobacillus* – added to feed.	Uses microbes as supplements to improve immunity to disease and speed of growth in chickens. Improved immune response, quicker growth.	Reduction in reliance on antibiotics because of impacts on antimicrobial resistance. Unchanged economic system.
	Beef	Adding a methanogenic – *3-Nitrooxypropanol* – to cattle feed.	Inhibiting microbes which produce methane leading to lower green house gas emissions from the herd.	Emissions reductions can be used to promote meat/dairy in diets.
	Cropping agriculture	Streptomyces, a bacteria known to be an important source of antibiotics, used as a seed coating.	Stimulates plant growth and protects against disease by competing with pathogens or inducing plant defences.	Reduced fertiliser and pesticide use and reduced pollution. Unchanged economic system.
Can be supplementary or transformative	Cropping agriculture	No-till or reduced-till to reduce the depth and frequency of tillage. Less disturbed soils are better able to host 'good' microbes.	Improves system connectivity through less breakage of beneficial fungal hyphae, improved soil health and carbon sequestration.	Reduced fertiliser usage and pollution. Potential need for increased herbicidal applications, particularly glyphosate. Also relevant to smaller farms.

(*Continued*)

TABLE 5.1 (Continued)

	Farm type	*Practice*	*Purposes*	*Repair through*
Transformative practices	Cropping agriculture	Agroecology: replace monocrop systems with diverse rotations of legumes, herbal leys etc. to encourage 'good' microbes.	Improved soil health, less reliance on chemical inputs to manage fertility and disease. 'Good' microbes help on both counts.	Higher rural employment. Greater seasonality and more traditional mixed farm practices. Risks of lower yields and knock-on impacts on food security.
	Mixed, cropping, or livestock agriculture	Agroforestry, silvo-pasture: use of trees and forestry to diversify production portfolio and create public goods. A more diverse ecosystem encourages microbe diversity.	Increased local biodiversity improved pest resistance (through microbes which compete with pathogens or induce host defences), increased carbon sequestration (via the action of microbes and other soil organisms).	Higher rural employment. Greater seasonality and more traditional mixed farm practices. Risks of lower yields and knock-on impacts on food security.

Biosocial practices of microbial repair: Attunement, co-cultivation and care

Attuning to dysbiosis

Our first set of probiotic farming practices emerge from an attunement to the implications of existing antibiotic approaches and involve paying attention to and making sensible previously invisible and neglected microbial worlds. Here farmers and researchers are changing the meaning of farming, re-imagining practices previously seen as human controlled and directed and viewing them as fundamentally biosocial. For example, drawing on the techniques (competencies) of microbiology, researchers have traced the role of microbes in the soil in fixing and mobilising nutrients to make them available to plant root systems (Suman et al., 2022). Others have examined the role of microbes in the stomachs of cattle, aiding in the digestion, metabolism and growth of livestock animals (Clemmons et al., 2019). But these new modes of attunement are not limited to microbiology. They also entail developing the skills and practical know-how – what Anna Tsing (2015) describes as 'arts of noticing' – required for working with a subset of often place- or terroir-specific microbes known to perform vital metabolic functions. These are most readily apparent in long established biosocial practices where humans and microbes work together in the production of foods such as artisan cheese production (Paxson, 2008), but they also – we contend – emerge in response to the challenges posed by antibiotic blowback.

A common refrain that runs through our ethnographic materials and which is echoed in influential published accounts (Brown, 2018; Tree, 2018) of microbial repair, is a moment of epiphany in which a farmer, agronomist or other agricultural expert realises, or finally accepts, the broken, dysfunctional or otherwise ruined nature of their land, herd, or personal bodily health. There is a point at which the harms done by an antibiotic mode of managing microbes, and the failure of modern methods for circumventing them, become undeniable. Such generative moments of blowback are diverse and include the persistent resistance of an infection to commonly used drugs, a dramatic crop failure in the context of declining yields, a moment of soil erosion, due to flooding or some other natural hazard. Sometimes these are experienced as an economic crisis: a bankruptcy or credit refusal. Sometimes they are felt through the sickness of animals, family members or air and water pollution. Often, they have an aesthetic register, a sense that the landscape or the animal does not look, sound or otherwise feel right, perhaps through a retrospective comparison to a time before.

Reflecting on these moments of crisis, practitioners talk of the scales falling away, and of a moment of revelation when they realised that they had been blinded or deceived by the logics of antibiotic agriculture. One large-scale commercial farmer in central England explained how a nascent interest in soil as the commercial underpinning of his farm business flourished into a full-bodied concern with the relationship between agrochemicals, human health and agroecological wellbeing:

> I wasn't aware of the impact the chemicals were having in our context… And then I suppose I started to become more aware of the poisonous impact of the pesticides, and then there was one event on the farm where I went out spraying... and I just remember being horrified by that, and then realising that actually I was probably giving a death sentence to the guy who's driving the sprayer normally.

In this way, farmers sense problems, developing new competencies in attuning to the ruined nature of the landscapes, bodies and ecologies in and through which they work. This leads to a shift in the way they understand farming. Farmers describe feelings of shame about the legacies of past modes of agriculture, grief as to what has been lost and an apprehension for the future. They question the practices to which they had become accustomed – for example of tilling, spraying, injecting or draining. They report how they decided (or were compelled by a change of economic circumstance) to 'step off the treadmill' of agrochemical application and fossil-fuelled acceleration.

Often this transition happens across generations, as the farm is handed on to a younger son or daughter, who may have been trained in different approaches to farming, and/or been infused with ecological values (or meanings) alien to their parents. Here, a young farmer who had recently returned to her family farm after years of study and working abroad, explains why her father had been so receptive to taking her advice about the management of soil's agroecological microbial health. The discussion here refers to a newly pesticide-resistant 'blackgrass' weed, and the farm's susceptibility to it owing to a recent legacy of intensive soil-depleting management:

> Blackgrass is a much more dominant issue for us. He is very aware that our costs are quite high… And he has been really open to ideas… When he first came back to the farm, his father was quite good for letting him lead the way, so I think he is trying quite hard to let me have a go.

Here there is a moment of disjuncture in which habituated practices and the biosocial norms – or perhaps more accurately antibiosocial norms – associated with them are brought into question as new practices and understandings of the biosocial relations cultivated through and with them emerge.

Co-cultivation

A second set of biosocial practices (more akin to those set out in Table 5.1) relate to how farmers adapt their land management as they shift from a chemical to a biological understanding of soil and begin to come to terms with the importance of the microbiome and the roles of beneficial microbes. Microbial repair is predicated on new approaches to microbiology, and to knowledge practices that have given rise to a new ontology for agriculture that understands health as a multispecies and ecological achievement. This first involves a shift in meanings away from the logics of chemistry that predominate modern soil science and agronomy, and towards the imaginaries of microbiology which understand and value microbes as a source of world-sustaining practices. The focus changes from a concern with the presence or absence of particular molecules (especially of nitrogen, phosphorus and potassium), towards the interactions of the fungi, bacteria and animals responsible for their production, decomposition, circulation and wider metabolism in the soil and on the farm (Barua, 2025).

Microbiome science remains an emerging field, and the agricultural implications of metagenomics and of the tools for understanding the metabolic functions of different microbes are not yet fully understood (Fierer, 2017). Nonetheless, implicitly recognising how 'past and present complexes of practice "prefigure" the future, making some trajectories more likely than others' (Shove et al., 2024), some probiotic pioneers have begun to develop competencies in sensing the soil (and other key agricultural microbiomes) to make them accessible to farmers and other publics. Microbiome research suggests that biodiverse-rich soils have positive impacts which ripple out across entire landscapes (Bardgett and Van Der Putten, 2014), that healthy soils create nutritionally dense foodstuffs (Montgomery et al., 2022), and that livestock antibiotic use shapes human exposure to antimicrobial resistance. Crucially, this approach draws attention to the pathological consequences of microbial absence, as well as to the (sometimes excessive) presence of specific microbes, showing that the loss of 'keystone' organisms can lead to the deleterious loss of function (suggesting some microbial practices are more valued or significant than others), as well as generating hotspots for the emergence of new pathogens (Schlatter et al., 2017).

While insights into very specific microbes are helping to produce generic and scalable inputs like biopesticides and biofertilisers, the repair of the microbiome calls for greater attention to be paid to site-specific needs. Owing to the complexity and variability of the microbiome, particularly in agricultural soils, in the agricultural sector there is now widespread acceptance that a given intervention is liable to lead to very different outcomes in different contexts (Fierer, 2017). There is, to put it differently, a recognition that microbiomes of different soils, animals, and plants need different things to be repaired well (Papadimitriou et al., 2015; Ray et al., 2020). Here, a soil scientist and hydrologist working for an agronomy research firm explain why farmers are increasingly expecting tailored advice sensitive to the microbial specifics of their land:

> Every farm's landscape is different. You could go, oh, like minimum till is great for reducing nitrous emissions from soil on that farm, but not that farm. But that's just one example about land type. So it's responding to the whole [...] one-size-fits-all approach.

Techniques for co-cultivating with microbes have also been pioneered by farmers and agronomists seeking to engage others in discussions of soil health, especially those involved in the vibrant movement towards regenerative agriculture that has grown substantially in the past decade (Granjou and Phillips, 2019). These modes of co-cultivating with microbes are also present in emerging practices of agroecology, which require farmers to engage with the spatiotemporal dynamics of their farm. A desire to work with the agricultural microbiome informs circular, multi-seasonal, and otherwise more complex models for choreographing agricultural practices that move away from the simplified, accelerated and linear temporalities of the antibiotic model (Cusworth and Lorimer, 2024).

For example, proponents of regenerative agriculture have been revisiting and reinventing sequences of crop rotation that were common before the invention of artificial fertilisers. They now fold together legumes, leys (permitting animal grazing for a season), and a heterogenous array of crops to build soil quantity and enhance fertility (Cusworth et al., 2021). Likewise, advocates of integrated pest management seeks to tackle outbreaks of drug-resistant microbes, plants and insects by choreographing ploughing, planting and harvesting cycles to encourage forms of biological control and pest suppression, working with microbes and other critters (Cusworth and Lorimer, 2024). In these contexts, the impulse towards notions of *diversity* and *crop diversification* figure both as a management heuristic and as an ideological rejection of the spatiotemporal simplification of antibiotic farm management ideals. As one farmer explained:

> It's time and place, time and space. When we grow a cover crop, we're adding diversity in that space. So, we've got an eleven way mix this year, and our herbal lays, you know, that's twelve or thirteen different species in there.

In this way a shift in meaning, specifically the reframing of soil health as a multispecies and ecological achievement, is supported by the development of new competencies in understanding local soil configurations (as microbially specific) and more complex models for choreographing agricultural practices (for example crop rotation) which in turn generate distinctive material configurations (such as crop diversification).

Collective care

A final bundle of practices emerges from the first two and involves farmers shaping new relationships of care that enact ethical relationships with the soil, crops and animals. These strategies recognise care as a collective, interdependent, symbiotic practice. This involves a revaluation of *who* (or what) is being cared for when one undertakes the work of microbial repair, and *with whom* the caring is being done. Farmers are recognising that to care for the soil well demands a proactive and pro-social approach to microbial repair; and that in caring for the soil, we are also caring for ourselves. As Henke and Sims note, a focus on practices of repair can act as 'an essential window into the ethics of care around socio-technical [and we would argue socio-natural] systems' (Henke and Sims, 2020:15). Here conceptions of an interconnected microbiome are co-produced alongside new ways of responding to the felt needs of a focal ecology. As various social scientists have documented, farmers becoming concerned with the soil develop new 'care-full' understandings of health beyond the human, concluding that the health of people is intrinsically linked to the microbial health of soils, plants and animals and the maintenance of connections through which beneficial microbes might be exchanged, through active touch and alongside the passive vectors of breathing air and drinking water (Krzywoszynska, 2019; Puig De La Bellacasa, 2015).

In other words, health is understood as a practical, multispecies and more-than-human achievement; a collective form of biosocial becoming which emerges through mundane practices of eating, cleaning (or dirtying) and healthcare. For example, health can be seen as the outcome of probiotic microbial exposure as a means of developing immunocompetency: Hinchliffe and Ward (2014) describe this process in their analysis of intensive pig farming and the ways in which farmers 'muck up' the sterile pigs that arrive on the farm with soil to help them build immunity.

Health is also a collective achievement. As our empirical studies show, practices of microbial repair entail, in the first instance, a softening of farmers' attitudes towards collective thought and action, and a breaking down of the individualistic mindset common to antibiotic intensive modes of management. Where the strictures of intensive and chemically dependent agriculture helped lead to the atomisation of rural society and the depopulation of farm labour, probiotic modes of management are emerging as knowledge-intensive systems that depend on social interaction. In the next extract, a regenerative farmer celebrates the emergence of *farm clusters*: collectives of farmers learning from each other's experiences of repair, both successful and otherwise:

> I think what we have to have is a bottom-up resurgence by people finding their own way forward by cluster group farming, by looking at what their neighbours are doing [...] then doing it themselves.

In this way the meanings, competencies and materials associated with microbial repair gain traction, expanding the human network of actors involved in the management and repair of the farm's agro-ecosystem. In the following quotation, a farmer explains how microbial absences in agricultural soil inveigle their way into the farm's accounting books:

> The people who have raped and pillaged their soils and their ecosystems ... they've got no pesticides to control all the rampant pests and things that have got out of control. And now they've got no fertilizers to put on the soil because there's no goodness in the soil, they won't have a functioning business.

This collective is evidently more-than-human. Reference to the *goodness in the soil* functions as a shorthand: a way of referring to soil's complex microbial configurations of bacteria, mycelia, worms, as well as balances of abiotic substances like moisture, aerated soil structure, organic matter, and bioavailable nutrients like nitrogen and phosphorus for plant growth. These ingredients allow the microbial needs of an agroecosystem to become a focal point of attention and care, even in the absence of comprehensive taxonomic knowledge of what that 'goodness' amounts to. Allusions to soil's *complexity* or its *goodness* encourage unnamed (and potentially unnameable) more-than-human constellations to become recipients of attention from both individual farmers and farmer collectives, as articulated by one of our interviewees:

> The composting process that goes on through the animal and all the biota that happens within the animal and the association of that with the soil base. That natural process, as they have done for hundreds and thousands of years, there's a symbiotic sort of relationship between grazing animals, soils, herbivores and plants.

In this way soils – as sites of microbial repair – serve as a nexus for the formation of practices of multispecies, collective, reciprocal care, which bundle together. These conjunctions include materials (such as compost and muck, moisture, soil structure and bioavailable nutrients) and infrastructures (such as farm clusters and untilled fields), meanings (such as an understanding of soil goodness, of microbes as lively allies as opposed to inert matter, and of health as collectively held and reproduced) and competencies (in carefully calibrated microbial exposures and soil care) – after Shove et al. (2012).

Discussion: The implications of biosocial repair

Having identified different bundles of biosocial practices which serve as routes to repair on the farm, in this section we reflect on what the lens of the biosocial brings to our understanding of the reconfiguration of human-microbe relations in probiotic – or what are often referred to as regenerative – farming practices.

Firstly, a key question running through this chapter is whether the reimagination of farming as a biosocial practice represents a move away from industrialised, intensive forms of agriculture. Some of the practices outlined in Table 5.1 involve very little change to established systems and infrastructures and often rely on substituting what we might term antibiotic interventions (including antibiotics and other technologies aimed at eradicating unwanted pests, weeds and pathogens) for probiotic ones in the form of novel biofertilisers, biopesticides, soil and feed additives. For example, using Lactobacillus (a probiotic supplement) as a feed additive for broiler chickens can improve the chickens' immune response and potentially reduce reliance on antibiotics in broiler systems, but involves very little change in terms of the scale or intensive nature of that agricultural system. In this case there is a shift in some of the materials used (probiotic additives), and to an extent in the meanings attributed to them, but the competencies required differ little from other forms of agriculture.

Other practices, however, require more significant, transformative, changes. For example, agroforestry involves the introduction of trees and forestry as part of a much more diverse, mixed farming system. This brings ecological benefits, including increased biodiversity, improved pest resistance and carbon sequestration, and entails wider social transformations, offering a source of rural employment and better engagement with seasonality, locality, and traditional mixed farm practices. Over time this work leads to the formation of new communities of practice.

The difference between these two kinds of biosocial practices suggests that repair can take different forms. On the one hand, supplementary biosocial practices align with types of repair concerned with the mundane maintenance of a system – often securing the status quo with a few microbes added for good measure. On the other hand, practices such as agroforestry are more transformative, seeking to fundamentally change biosocial arrangements in order to meet new challenges and/or redress past harms (Henke and Sims, 2020). Transformative biosocial repair has the potential to reconfigure the conceptual architecture of modern agronomy (predicated on neat divisions between isolated elements in a system) that defined a previous generation of agricultural research and development. It leads to new approaches to farming in response to an environment understood as emergent and shaped by the biosocial practices of humans and microbes.

Secondly, paying attention to farming practices invites reflection on the origins of these biosocial formations. In one sense the rise of probiotic farming in the West is seen as a break with (or at least questioning of) previous methods and with the knowledge of earlier generations. In this way, a focus on biosocial practices complements and extends previous work on microbiopolitics by paying close and careful attention to how farmers respond to the imperative to use life to manage life, not least through relinquishing at least some of the control (or at least the appearance of control) that dominated the agricultural sector. But there are also continuities, as farmers engaged in biosocial techniques draw inspiration (and meaning) from practices and systems that have evaded the dysbiosis that characterises forms of industrial agriculture. Their reinvention of the past is characterised by a focus on both materials-turned-biosocial-collaborators such as heritage crops and cultivars, soils, and animal breeds, and on competencies inspired by indigenous and traditional agricultural practices (Chen et al., 2021). In short, practices of microbial repair have antecedents, and while a sense of the biosocial may be novel in Western academia it has been a central feature of many different farming traditions over millennia.

Finally, a focus on the agricultural microbiome leads to a recognition of myriad ways in which biosocial practices connect and have effect at scale (Hui et al., 2016; Schatzki, 2016). Drawing attention to how social practice theory might engage with large phenomena, Schatzki suggests that 'kitchen arrangements directly link, causally and physically, with the arrangements that make up the power grid and also physically, though more indirectly, with the arrangements composing the grocery store and road system' (2016: 6). Geographers have also concluded that the interlinking of practices like cooking, shopping and farming creates a relational ethics which ties food production and consumption together through what Krzywoszynska terms a 'soil food-web model of care relations' (2019: 665) (see also Puig de la Bellacasa, 2015). As Roe describes, processes like eating a burger are replete with a series of social and environmental relations generated through the 'numerous practices that have brought it [the burger] into being, from artificial insemination, to meat processing techniques, and the skills of marketers' (Roe, 2010: 262). But, as Roe also notes, such extended networks of digestion and consumption pose challenges for allocating political and ethical responsibility with profound consequences for how the human is co-constituted (Roe, 2010: 277).

Following Henke and Sims (2020) we go along with the view that microbial repair practices are constituted by and constitutive of wider biosocial relations: past and present harms and benefits must also be on the agenda when we consider repair, and repair can refer to fixing relationships and understandings as well as technologies and infrastructures. This happens at the scale of individual farms, where practicing microbial care also requires a specific disposition, embodied in an ethos of stewardship, husbandry and co-cultivation. It also happens on a broader scale as those practicing microbial repair relate their work to broader questions of environmental and social justice (Cusworth et al., 2025). For example, whilst antimicrobial resistance might emerge (at least in part) from particular farming practices, its consequences extend far beyond the scale of individual farms (see Hinchliffe et al., 2018). Consequently, microbes, we suggest, act as both an index of the ways in which biosocial practices interact at scale, and as an indicator of the implications of these interactions for human, animal and environmental health.

Conclusion

Drawing on both lived experience and microbiological expertise, the farmers with whom we spoke described a shift in perspective – from seeing soils as inert substrates to valuing them as living matters in need of care, co-produced through relations with microbial allies and necessary to sustain human and environmental health. This may represent wider recognition of the view that farming is a biosocial practice. Secondly, some forms of industrial farming are moving away from the use of the use of agrochemical inputs and systems of intensive tillage and adopting practices which sustain soil health such as no-till systems, agroforestry and permaculture. Significantly, some farmers are rejecting the model of substitution (involving new but still intensive uses of land) and seeking to develop new competencies in attuning to and caring for soil health. This represents a radical break with the farming techniques of the previous generation, but a form of continuity with indigenous and traditional practice.

References

Bardgett, R. and Van Der Putten, W. (2014). 'Belowground biodiversity and ecosystem functioning', *Nature*, 515(7528): 505–511. https://doi.org/10.1038/nature13855.
Barua, M. (2025). 'Metabolic politics: A comparative synthesis', *Transactions of the Institute of British Geographers*, e12712. https://doi.org/10.1111/tran.12712.
Beck, A. (2021). 'Microbiomes as companion species: An exploration of dis- and re-entanglements with the microbial self', *Social and Cultural Geography*, 22(3): 357–375. https://doi.org/10.1080/14649365.2019.1593490.
Beck, U. (1992). *Risk Society: Towards a new modernity*. London: Sage Publications.
Brown, G. (2018). *Dirt to Soil: One family's journey into regenerative agriculture*. New York: Chelsea Green Publishing.

Chen, Q-L., Hu H-W., He, Z.-Y., Cui, L., Zhu, Y-G. and He, J-Z. (2021). 'Potential of indigenous crop microbiomes for sustainable agriculture', *Nature Food*, 2(4): 233–240. https://doi.org/10.1038/s43016-021-00253-5.

Clemmons B., Voy B. and Myer P. (2019). 'Altering the gut microbiome of cattle: Considerations of host-microbiome interactions for persistent microbiome manipulation', *Microbial Ecology*, 77(2): 523–536. https://doi.org/10.1007/s00248-018-1234-9.

Cusworth, G., Finlay, B., Nguyen, N. and Lorimer, J. (2025). 'Microbial repair and ecological justice: A new paradigm for agriculture', *npj Sustainable Agriculture*, 3(1): 23. https://doi.org/10.1038/s44264-025-00062-4.

Cusworth, G., Garnett, T. and Lorimer J. (2021). 'Agroecological break out: Legumes, crop diversification and the regenerative futures of UK agriculture', *Journal of Rural Studies*, 88: 126–137. https://doi.org/10.1016/j.jrurstud.2021.10.005.

Cusworth, G., Lorimer, J., Brice, J. and Garnett, T. (2022). 'Green rebranding: Regenerative agriculture, future-pasts, and the naturalisation of livestock', *Transactions of the Institute of British Geographers*, 47(4): 1009–1027. https://doi.org/10.1111/tran.12555.

Cusworth, G. and Lorimer J. (2024). 'On disease configurations, black-grass blowback, and probiotic pest management', *Annals of the American Association of Geographers*, 114(3): 462–480. https://doi.org/10.1080/24694452.2023.2289984.

Fierer, N. (2017). 'Embracing the unknown: Disentangling the complexities of the soil microbiome', *Nature Reviews Microbiology*, 15(10): 579–590. https://doi.org/10.1038/nrmicro.2017.87.

Frąc, M., Hannula, M., Bełka, M., Salles, J. and Jedryczka, M. (2022). 'Soil mycobiome in sustainable agriculture', *Frontiers in Microbiology*, 13. https://doi.org/10.3389/fmicb.2022.1033824.

Granjou, C. and Phillips, C. (2019). 'Living and labouring soils: Metagenomic ecology and a new agricultural revolution?', *BioSocieties*, 14(3): 393–415. https://doi.org/10.1057/s41292-018-0133-0.

Hartmann, M. and Six, J. (2023). 'Soil structure and microbiome functions in agroecosystems', *Nature Reviews Earth and Environment*, 4(1): 4–18. https://doi.org/10.1038/s43017-022-00366-w.

Henke C. and Sims, B. (2020). *Repairing Infrastructures: The maintenance of materiality and power*. Cambridge MA: MIT Press.

Hinchliffe S., Butcher, A. and Rahman M. (2018). 'The AMR problem: demanding economies, biological margins, and co-producing alternative strategies', *Palgrave Commun*, 4, 142.

Hinchliffe, S. and Ward, K. (2014). 'Geographies of folded life: How immunity reframes biosecurity', *Geoforum*, 53: 136–144. https://doi.org/10.1016/j.geoforum.2014.03.002.

Hui A., Schatzki T., and Shove, E. (eds.). (2016). *The Nexus of Practices: Connections, constellations, practitioners*. London: Routledge. https://doi.org/10.4324/9781315560816.

Krzywoszynska, A. (2019). 'Caring for soil life in the Anthropocene: The role of attentiveness in more-than-human ethics', *Transactions of the Institute of British Geographers*, 44(4), 661–675. https://doi.org/10.1111/tran.12293.

Lehmann J., Bossio D., Kögel-Knabner I., and Rillig, M. (2020). 'The concept and future prospects of soil health', *Nat Rev Earth Environ*, 1(10): 544–553. https://doi.org/10.1038/s43017-020-0080-8.

Lorimer, J. (2020). *The Probiotic Planet: Using life to manage life*. Minneapolis: University of Minnesota Press. https://doi.org/10.5749/j.ctv19cw9vg.
Montgomery, D., Biklé, A., Archuleta, R., Brown, P. and Jordan, J. (2022). 'Soil health and nutrient density: Preliminary comparison of regenerative and conventional farming', *PeerJ*, 10: e12848. https://doi.org/10.7717/peerj.12848.
Montgomery, D., Rabinowitz, P., Sipos, Y. and Wheat, E. (2024). 'Soil health: A common focus for one health and planetary health interventions', *One Health*, 18: 100673. https://doi.org/10.1016/j.onehlt.2023.100673.
Nasem – National Academies of Sciences, Engineering, and Medicine (2024). *Exploring linkages between soil health and human health*. Special Report by National Academies of Sciences, Engineering and Medicine. Washington, US. Available at: www.nationalacademies.org/read/27459.
Papadimitriou, K., Zoumpopoulou, B., Foligné, V., Alexandraki, M., Kazou, B., Pot, B. and Tsakalidou, E. (2015). 'Discovering probiotic microorganisms: In vitro, in vivo, genetic and omics approaches' *Frontiers in Microbiology*, 6(1): 1–12. https://doi.org/10.3389/fmicb.2015.00058.
Paxson, H. (2008). 'Post-pasteurian cultures: The microbiopolitics of raw-milk cheese in the united states', *Cultural Anthropology*, 23(1): 15–47. https://doi.org/10.1111/j.1548-1360.2008.00002.x.
Paxson, H. and Helmreich, S. (2014). 'The perils and promises of microbial abundance: Novel natures and model ecosystems, from artisanal cheese to alien seas', *Social Studies of Science*, 44(2): 165–193. https://doi.org/10.1177/0306312713505003.
Puig De La Bellacasa, M. (2015). 'Making time for soil: Technoscientific futurity and the pace of care', *Social Studies of Science*, 45(5): 691–716. https://doi.org/10.1177/0306312715599851.
Ray, P., Lakshmanan, V., Labbé, J., and Craven, K. (2020). 'Microbe to microbiome: A paradigm shift in the application of microorganisms for sustainable agriculture', *Frontiers in Microbiology*, 11(1): 1–25. https://doi.org/10.3389/fmicb.2020.622926.
Roe, E. (2010). 'Ethics and the non-human: The matterings of animal sentience in the meat industry' in Harrison, P. (ed.) *Taking-place: Non-representational theories and geography*. Aldershot: Ashgate Publishing.
Schatzki, T. (2002). *The Site of the Social: A philosophical account of the constitution of social life and change*, Pennsylvania: Penn State University Press.
Schatzki, T. (2016). 'Keeping track of large phenomena', *Geographische Zeitschrift*, 104(1): 4–24.
Schlatter, D., Kinkel, L., Thomashow, L., Weller, D. and Paulitz, T. (2017). 'Disease suppressive soils: New insights from the soil microbiome', *Phytopathology*, 107(11): 1284–1297. https://doi.org/10.1094/PHYTO-03-17-0111-RVW.
Shove, E., Blue, S. and Kelly M.P. (2024). 'Categorising and cohabiting: Practices as the site of biosocial becoming', *Social Theory and Health*, 22(2): 156–171. https://doi.org/10.1057/s41285-024-00204-7.
Shove, E., Pantzar, M. and Watson, M. (2012). *The Dynamics of Social Practice: Everyday life and how it changes*. London: Sage. https://doi.org/10.4135/9781446250655.
Singh, B., Trivedi, P., Egidi, E., Macdonald, C. and Delgado-Baquerizo, M. (2020). 'Crop microbiome and sustainable agriculture'. *Nature Reviews Microbiology*, 18(11): 601–602.

Suman, J., Rakshit, A., Ogireddy, S., Singh, S., Gupta, C. and Chandrakala, J. (2022). 'Microbiome as a key player in sustainable agriculture and human health'. *Frontiers in Soil Science*, 2. https://doi.org/10.1038/s41579-020-00446-y.

Tree, I. (2018). *Wilding: The return of nature to a British farm.* London: Pan Macmillan.

Tsing, A. (2015). *The Mushroom at the End of the World: On the possibility of life in capitalist ruins.* Princeton NJ: Princeton University Press.

Van Den Bosch, R. (1978). *The Pesticide Conspiracy.*, New York: Doubleday.

Wallace, R. and Wallace, R. G., (2015). 'Blowback: New formal perspectives on agriculturally driven pathogen evolution and spread', *Epidemiology and Infection*, 143(10): 2068–2080. https://doi.org/10.1017/S0950268814000077.

Woolhouse, M., Ward, M., Van Bunnik, B., and Farrar, J., (2015). 'Antimicrobial resistance in humans, livestock and the wider environment', *Philosophical Transactions of the Royal Society B: Biological Sciences*, 370(1670): 20140083. https://doi.org/10.1098/rstb.2014.0083.

Zhang, A. (2024). *Circular Ecologies: Environmentalism and waste politics in urban China.* Redwood City CA: Stanford University Press.

6

HOLOBIONT PUBLIC HEALTH?

Changing practices of allergy prevention in Finland

Mikko Jauho

Introduction

Microbiome science has triggered a paradigm shift in biology and medicine, fundamentally altering human relationships with microbes from a primarily adversarial perspective to a recognition of them as essential partners in health. A common way to describe this shift is to distinguish between established antiseptic (or antibiotic) and emerging probiotic paradigms (Paxson, 2013; Lorimer, 2020). The former foregrounds microbial pathology and purity and frames microbes as invisible enemies that need to be contained and eradicated, whereas the latter stresses microbial ecology and diversity and regards microbes as vital companions whose co-existence must be respected. Once viewed principally as pathogens, microorganisms are now understood to be critical components of human development, functioning and health.

One of my aims is to explore the impact of this paradigm shift on public health. Cutting-edge microbiome science has produced novel insights regarding the ecological underpinnings of (human) health and generated a call for a holobiont practice of public health (Sariola and Gilbert, 2020). Holobiont is a concept from biology that refers to a host organism and all its associated microorganisms, which together form a single ecological unit. The term emphasises the interconnectedness and interdependence of the host and its microbiome, recognising that they function as a complex, integrated whole rather than as separate entities. Considering the human body as an ecosystem involves reevaluating how we approach health and disease. Health is no longer primarily an individual attribute but an 'emergent property of a network of relationships' (Raffaetà, 2023: 1). A holobiont approach to public health shifts the focus from treating diseases in isolation to promoting overall

DOI: 10.4324/9781003685210-8

ecosystem health, recognising the dynamic relationship between humans and the myriad microorganisms with which they co-exist.

I therefore discuss the adoption of holobiont ideas into current public health strategies, particularly focusing on allergy prevention in Finland. Science has involved the microbiome in processes ranging from digestion and metabolism to immune system development, and alterations in microbial communities have been associated with an array of complex diseases, including metabolic disorders such as obesity, diabetes, cardiovascular diseases as well as neurological, inflammatory, and oncological conditions (Van Hul and Cani, 2026). Allergic diseases in Finland are a particularly salient case from public health perspective. In the current biomedical understanding, a lack of exposure to microbial diversity during early life contributes to allergies and other conditions (Haahtela, 2019). This 'biodiversity hypothesis' has been significantly developed in Finland (Haahtela et al., 2021) and is currently being adopted in public health strategies. The Finnish allergy landscape thus presents an excellent example through which to examine the impact of microbiome science and the role of holobionts in mainstream public health.

For this study, I draw from practice theory, which analyses shared, routinised activities as the primary unit of social life (Shove et al., 2012). Present public health measures form 'a complex of connected and co-dependent practices that take place in common settings or locations, carried out with a certain logic and order' (Maller, 2018: 118). Public health measures both target certain everyday practices as important for health and themselves represent specific policy practices. As I show, these sets of practices constrain and channel the way microbial allergy prevention is being introduced into mainstream public health.

The chapter begins with two sections that contrast heuristically the antiseptic (or antibiotic) and probiotic approach to microbes. Drawing on Latour (1988), who famously asserted that the discovery of microbes changed society, I then ask, how is the new, probiotic understanding of microbes affecting public health. After introducing the concept of holobiont public health and practice theory, the next three sections focus on allergy, the biodiversity hypothesis and microbial strategies against allergy, showing how new preventive methods rely on well-established practices. The conclusion underscores the importance of understanding the practices that condition the realisation of more-than-human health visions, and serves as an antidote to overly-enthusiastic narratives of revolutionary change often associated with microbiome science.

Classic hygiene and an antiseptic approach to microbes

In *The Pasteurization of France*, Bruno Latour (1988) examines how microbes became central to public health, focusing on the efforts of Louis

Pasteur in advancing bacteriology. Latour argues that Pasteur secured his status by leveraging the laboratory to address societal issues related to public health, agriculture and food production, building alliances with politicians, medical professionals, industrialists and agriculturalists. The alignment of Pasteur's work with the interests of these groups facilitated the widespread acceptance of microbes as central to public health and other concerns.

Latour identifies hygienists as Pasteur's key allies. These experts in preventive public health initially attributed diseases' spread to miasmas – noxious odours arising from decaying matter and filth. Consequently, their approach to health improvement focused on environmental sanitation, such as building sewage systems, ensuring clean water supply and promoting urban cleanliness. However, these measures failed to consistently explain and effectively control infectious disease outbreaks. Microbial theory provided a solution by shifting the focus from indirect preventive measures to targeted interventions addressing harmful bacteria.

In Latour's science of associations, new actants change society. Pasteur and his followers made previously invisible microbial worlds visible and thus 'redefined the social link by including the action of the microbes in it' (Latour, 1988: 38). Pasteurians were positioned as exclusive interpreters of this domain. This empowerment not only increased their influence but transformed societal practices by incorporating microbial presence as a factor in various fields.

However, according to Latour, hygienists usually conceived of microbial presence in negative terms. Microbes disrupted social processes, damaging food quality, souring wine, inflaming wounds, etc. The hygienists' challenge was to 'divert the microbes so that they will no longer intervene in relations everywhere' (Latour, 1988: 39). Destroy the microbes, and social relations become pure: 'if we wish to obtain economic and social relations in the strict sense, we must first extirpate the microbe. But in order to extirpate the microbe, we must place the representatives of the hygienists or Pasteurians everywhere' (Latour, 1988: 39). Thus, hygienists were tasked not only with interpreting the new microbial world but also acting as its stewards. They promoted an *antiseptic approach* to microbes, which defined microbes as sources of infection and contamination, necessitating control and cleanliness as essential responses.

Microbiome science and probiotic microbes

The currently emerging understanding of microbes in health and other matters can be compared to the transformative insights of bacteriology at the turn of the 20th century. In this case, the contemporary constellation is no longer about bacteriology but metagenomics, microbiomes, and ecological microbial diversity. Microbial species and singularised pathogens are now being reassessed from this perspective, and from a position that draws on an environmental tradition of microbiology and that focuses on microbial action in natural metabolism instead of pathogenic microbes (Rosenberg and Zilber-Rosenberg, 2013).

According to Raffaetà (2023), a key impetus for this new microbial knowledge emerged from the Human Genome Project (HGP) (1993–2000), the aim of which was to map the entire human genome, thereby unlocking the secrets of human functioning and health and paving the way for biomedical innovation. Originally, the HGP was underpinned by the belief that genes were autonomous entities capable of shaping an organism's biological outcomes in a straightforward manner. However, contemporary epigenetics has shifted this perspective, emphasising complex and dynamic interactions between genes and diverse environmental factors – from molecular to social stimuli – that have the 'capacity to modulate the information contained in the genome itself in the course of an individual's life' (Raffaetà, 2023: 41). Thus, in this model, the environment directly influences gene activity and, in some cases, heritable traits within one or two generations.

Technological advances associated with the HGP provided the scientific community with powerful genetic sequencing tools which have become faster and more cost-efficient over time. These developments have enabled scientists to analyse genetic content from samples sourced directly from specific environments, thereby generating data on microorganisms previously inaccessible through traditional methods of isolation and cultivation. This new data-intensive approach, known as metagenomics, has illuminated the immense diversity and ubiquity of microbes everywhere. Metagenomics analyses the genomes of microbial communities, or microbiomes, that populate specific locations. The human microbiome refers to 'the ecological community of commensal, symbiotic, and pathogenic microorganisms that [...] share our body space' (Lederberg and McCray, 2001: 8). It is now understood that microbial cells are nearly equal in number to human cells, with microbial genes vastly outnumbering human ones (Sender et al., 2016).

These scientific findings have led to profound changes in how we perceive living entities, the environment, and their interrelationships, all of which involve microbes. First, humans and other living entities are understood as holobionts, metaorganisms that consist of the host and the associated microbiome. Organisms are complex entities with evolving symbiotic relationships with microbes, which are considered integral to the health and functioning of bodies and ecosystems. Second, epigenetics has changed our understanding of organisms' adaptability to environmental changes. Microbes react to human activity, the effects of which are impressed on and recorded in microbial lives. For example, the pervasive use of antibiotics, disinfectants and heavy metals have exerted selection pressures that encourage the emergence of microbial variants with drug-resistant genes, causing antimicrobial resistance

(Landecker, 2016). Lateral gene transfer further accelerates these adaptations by facilitating genetic material exchange not only between generations but also among adjacent microbial species. Third, modern environments have been rendered increasingly sterile due to pervasive sanitation practices, leading to the removal of spontaneous and unpredictable natural elements (Sariola and Gilbert, 2020). This leads to critical absences of microbes in environments that are vital for health, such as soil and the human gut. These 'missing microbes' (Blaser, 2014) are identified as the cause of 'epidemics of absence' (Velasquez-Manoff, 2012), characterised by dysbiosis and disrupted symbiotic relations. The classic hygiene practices designed to manage and control microbial threats have, paradoxically, generated new pathologies.

According to Lorimer (2020), these insights have fostered a new *probiotic sensibility* towards living entities and processes. This sensibility 'links a range of efforts that aim to change the composition of biophysical systems to modulate the rhythms and intensities of their ecological interactions. These [...] projects control, restore and enhance the functioning of ecosystems to secure a desired set of systemic properties – [for example] – biodiversity and immunity.' This represents a transition from an antiseptic or antibiotic mindset to a probiotic, 'post-Pasteurian' approach to microbes that is 'committed to working in selective partnership with microscopic organisms, figured as agents of a nature that is not fully objectified and never fully separate from human enterprise' (Paxson, 2013: 161). While antibiotic strategies are designed to kill or inhibit harmful bacteria, probiotic strategies focus on supporting, replenishing and fostering beneficial microbes to maintain balanced, healthy microbial ecosystems.

The opposition should not be understood as a historical break, a movement from an antiseptic (or antibiotic) to a probiotic age. Probiotic relationships with microbes existed in the early 20th century (e.g. fermentation in food production), and antibiotic strategies are still prominent. However, there is a change of emphasis, with new interest in opportunities associated with microbes and in the problems caused by their absence. The presence of microbes is no longer (only) a negative factor, disturbing social life, but is also defined as vital to the thriving of social and ecological relations. Therefore, the insights leveraged by the science of the microbiome can be seen to create an analogous situation to the one described by Latour. Like his Pasteurians, post-Pasteurian microbiome scientists and public health advocates are redefining the social link: not by introducing a novel actant but by reconceptualising an existing one and its associations.

Holobiont public health and how to approach it

How might the probiotic shift impact public health practices? What new associations are microbes implicated in when holobiont public health is advocated? There is an on-going discussion on the precarious state of ecological systems and the ecological underpinnings of (human) health. From this two-way problematisation of health and ecology has emerged an ecological concept of public health, which posits that health arises from intricate interactions between individuals and their environments (Mallee, 2017).

The ecological concept of public health has developed through various frameworks that exhibit increasingly complex conceptions of the natural environment (Coutts et al., 2014). Environmental medicine, rooted in the sanitary spirit of classic public hygiene, primarily focuses on environmental health hazards and safety in urban contexts. Social ecological models frame ecology as a multi-level construct that encompasses intrapersonal, interpersonal, organisational, community and policy levels (McLeroy et al., 1988), defining the natural environment as one of several factors that shape health behaviours and outcomes (Hancock 1993). Health promotion efforts often adopt this perspective, fostering environments that encourage healthy behaviours in individuals (Patja et al., 2022). More advanced iterations of the ecological paradigm, including conservation medicine (Aguirre et al., 2002), EcoHealth, One Health, and Planetary Health (Lerner and Berg, 2017), treat the natural environment not as an external factor but as a dynamic, interconnected system fundamental to human health. This encompasses both the adverse health effects of environmental degradation and the benefits derived from interactions with nature.

The probiotic, post-Pasteurian understanding of microbes gives ecological public health a specific microbial inflection. It calls for 'a holobiont practice of public health' that recognises 'the webs of symbioses uniting different species of organisms into a collective "individual" and uniting these different individual teams into complex ecosystems' (Sariola and Gilbert, 2020: 746). In this 'ecosystemic perspective of health' (Raffaetà, 2023: 44).

> Health is no longer described as the property of an organism whose immune system works to repulse and kill enemy invaders. We have entered an era where we are told that interrelating with a myriad of microbes is not only unavoidable but necessary and that it lies at the basis of our wellbeing. We can thus begin to think of organisms as ecosystems and, consequently, of health as the emergent property of a dynamic ecosystem with permeable boundaries, rather than as a property of single bodies.
>
> *(Raffaetà, 2023: 3-4)*

Holobiont public health conceptualises health in terms of a complex, integrated, ecological system comprising the host and its microbiome, the holobiont. Health is contingent upon a fine-tuned equilibrium within this system and disruptions, or dysbiosis, can lead to various diseases and disorders. Ecological interactions significantly influence the holobiont's health, highlighting the need for a healthy external environment (e.g. urban biodiversity) to support beneficial microbiota necessary for bodily functions and immune development. This approach shifts the focus of public health from treating diseases or preventing illness in isolated individuals to managing the entire holobiont system in its ecological situation.

Although approaches such as One Health and Planetary Health are institutionalised and supported by departments, societies and journals, it remains unclear how these models are being adopted into mainstream public health arrangements. I will explore emerging holobiont methods through a case study of allergy control in Finland, a country in which a microbially-mediated environmental approach to addressing allergies is both scientifically explored and practically implemented.

To achieve this goal, it is helpful to approach public health through the lens of *social practices*. The term 'practice theory' refers to a family of theories that share the premise that practices are the foundational units for investigating social life (Reckwitz, 2002). Instead of starting from individuals and their attitudes, behaviours and choices, practice theory focuses on social practices, defined as patterned habitual doings and sayings that extend across time and space (Shove et al., 2012). Social practices are characterised by routine and repetition but are dynamic and changing due to modulations introduced by practitioners when performing the practice. Practices are also shaped by material arrangements and infrastructures (e.g., urban design, transportation systems and housing) (Shove and Trentmann, 2018) and interconnected, forming larger conglomerates, bundles and complexes (Hui et al., 2017). A prominent way to parse social practices is to define them with the help of three interconnected elements: materials, meanings and know-how (Shove et al., 2012). Stressing the materiality of social practices is a key aspect of what Maller calls the 'second wave of the practice tradition' (Maller, 2018: 73) originating from Schatzki, Shove and colleagues. Recently, 'a post-humanist subset of The Practice Turn' (Maller, 2018: 11) has extended this interest in materiality to 'dynamic non-humans' (Strengers and Maller, 2018), which include animals, plants, robots and microbes.

From the perspective of practice theory, 'health is the product of participation in entire sets of practices, complexes and bundles' (Maller, 2018: 100). Thus, public health policy must 'focus on the "lives" of social practices, treating social practices as topics of analysis and as sites of intervention in their own right' (Blue et al., 2016: 38). In this spirit, research inspired by practice theory has discussed various health topics, such as smoking (Blue et al., 2016; Maller, 2015), obesity (Blue et al., 2021), and urban health challenges (Maller, 2018), showcasing the value of practice theory as an analytical lens for reframing public health issues. These studies often address policy actors and programme deliverers, denouncing existing approaches and offering alternative definitions and measures of intervention informed by practice theory. Practice theory scholars have been especially critical of two prevalent models of public health (Blue et al., 2016). One is psychological theories of behaviour change that emphasise individuals' knowledge, attitudes and choices in promoting healthy habits. These methods make individuals responsible for their health and overestimate their capacity for self-regulation (see also Shove, 2010). The other includes structural approaches that investigate health inequalities or the social determinants of health, but often 'fail to show exactly how these translate into the daily lives (and hence health) of different sectors of the population' (Blue et al., 2016: 36).

In this chapter, I am interested in the public health models to which holobiont ideas are attached. Moreover, I will discuss the everyday practices that are implicitly involved in allergy prevention in these models. On both levels I focus on continuity and change, and on how existing practices of public health influence the incorporation of innovative approaches in microbial allergy prevention and holobiont public health.

Allergy and the biodiversity hypothesis

Biomedicine defines allergy as an exaggerated immune response by the body to an otherwise innocuous environmental substance, such as specific foods, pollen or dust to which the individual has become hypersensitive. Current diagnostic practices comprise prick tests on the skin and blood tests that measure allergen-specific IgE antibodies. Allergic diseases encompass a heterogeneous group of conditions, including allergic rhinitis and conjunctivitis, asthma, atopic dermatitis and allergies to foods, drugs and insect stings. From the holobiont perspective, allergies are often associated with autoimmune diseases such as rheumatoid arthritis and type 1 diabetes, as both categories involve immune system malfunctions (see Haahtela, 2019).

The global prevalence of allergic diseases has increased to epidemic proportions after WW2 (Platts-Mills, 2015), with a notable rise also observed in Finland (Latvala et al., 2005). Several theories have been proposed to explain this trend, ranging from greater exposure to environmental pollutants and chemicals to dietary shifts, such as increased consumption of processed foods and changes in fat consumption.

One significant stream of hypotheses with a pronounced microbial component focuses on environmental interactions in contemporary urbanised settings. The hygiene hypothesis (Strachan, 1989) argues that decreased exposure to infections during early childhood – attributable to improved hygiene practices and smaller family sizes – has contributed to a heightened susceptibility to allergic diseases. The 'old friends' hypothesis (Rook et al., 2004) extends this narrative by suggesting that modern lifestyles have diminished exposure to important evolutionary companions, such as microbes and parasites, which has led to immune system dysregulation and allergy development.

A notable extension of this discourse is the biodiversity hypothesis, which posits that contact with rich natural environments and beneficial microbial diversity reduces the risk of allergies and autoimmune diseases, and that modern living environments and lifestyles often jeopardise such contact (Haahtela, 2019). From this perspective, biodiversity enriches the human microbiome, trains the immune system to differentiate between harmful and harmless entities, and promotes immune balance. This view has a strong 'family resemblance' to the other hypotheses just outlined but differs from them in its ecological bent and stronger focus on natural environments and biodiversity.

The biodiversity hypothesis evolved from Finnish allergology, which has acquired a specific ecological characteristic. It was articulated by Tari Haahtela, a leading figure in the field of allergology in Finland, together with the population ecologist Ilkka Hanski and other collaborators, synthesising insights from immunology, microbiome research and ecology (von Hertzen et al., 2011; Hanski et al., 2012). The hypothesis was informed by comparative studies conducted by Haahtela's team in Finnish and Russian Karelia – two geo-climatically similar areas with genetically comparable populations but where significant health disparities corresponded to differences in microbial exposure. In Finland, high levels of hygiene correlated with increased allergy prevalence, while just across the border, a rich microbial habitat appeared to offer protection against these conditions (Haahtela et al., 2015). Similar results have been reported from other countries (see von Mutius et al., 1992). These insights subsequently guided the Finnish Allergy Programme (2008–2018), which Haahtela led. Prior prevention strategies emphasised the importance of avoiding allergens based on the premise that sensitisation necessitated prior exposure. The national programme shifted the focus towards restoring and strengthening tolerance, positing that too much protection from early exposure could be counterproductive. This shift was justified by the perceived failure of the old approach and bolstered by findings that support the biodiversity hypothesis (Haahtela et al., 2021).

Forwarding the biodiversity hypothesis

Current developments in the Finnish allergy field are reinforcing the biodiversity hypothesis. A new regional pilot programme, Nature Step to Health (2022–2032) deepens the environmental focus of the previous National Allergy Programme. It seeks to enhance both human and ecological health by promoting healthy lifestyles and sustainable urban development in the Lahti region (a middle-sized city in Southern Finland) (Hämäläinen et al.,

2023). The new National Nature Health Programme (2026–2035) aims to 'increase well-being and reduce chronic diseases by strengthening exposure to nature' (Halonen et al. 2026: 6) Initiatives by the Finnish Lung Health Association and by the Allergy, Skin and Asthma Federation also attest to the influence of the biodiversity hypothesis on stakeholders across national, regional and third-sector levels in Finland. These programmes focus on prevention and suppose that contact with nature is a crucial aspect of health and well-being in relation to allergic conditions and beyond.

In the realm of research, a multidisciplinary team in Finland is actively adding to the biodiversity hypothesis and integrating biomedical and ecological insights.[1] One principal research objective is to provide robust biomedical evidence of the public health benefits associated with increased microbial contact. Small clinical trials have already suggested the positive effects of dwelling in microbially rich environments on the microbiota of the mouth, skin, and gut, relevant immunological biomarkers (Roslund et al., 2022), and on perceived well-being (Puhakka et al., 2019). Two larger ongoing trials involve infants with strong family histories of autoimmune diseases (allergy, asthma or atopy) and older children in kindergarten settings.[2] Positive results from these trials would significantly reinforce the legitimacy of promoting microbial contact within allergy prevention initiatives and further bolster holobiont ideas in public health.

Other research focuses on human-environmental relationships that affect the commensal microbiome. This work investigates the mechanisms of environmental impact on microbiomes and the characteristics of environments that are favourable for such impact. Studies have begun to explore factors that influence the natural transfer of outdoor microbes indoors, such as pets or land use around homes (Parajuli et al., 2018), as well as the effects on microbiomes when natural elements, such as green walls (Soininen et al., 2022) and gardening (Saarenpää et al., 2024), are introduced in indoor environments. Recent work has also examined the microbial compositions of various environmental types and plant taxa (Roslund et al., 2024) with the aim of identifying settings rich in health-promoting microbial biodiversity. Collectively these studies lay the groundwork for strategies of 'immunomodulatory urban greening' (Soininen et al., 2024: 1) to be utilised in the development of green areas for public health purposes.

A noteworthy outgrowth of this research is the development of new products designed to promote microbial health benefits. One innovation is the creation of durable landscaping materials that contain microbial communities resembling the forest environment. These materials can be used in specific locations, like kindergarten yards, to help remediate soil contamination and support the immune system (Soininen et al., 2024). Another significant product is a patented soil- and plant-based microbial extract dubbed Reconnecting Nature™, designed to be placed in everyday consumer items to provide safe beneficial microbial exposure (see Hui et al., 2019). The extract consists of 'inactivated' microbes, which cannot reproduce but which retain their immunological properties. It is produced by a spin-off company, Uute Scientific, which licenses it for commercial use. Though utilised on a limited scale, the extract has already been incorporated into various household products, including baby clothes, cosmetics and items for pets.

Practices and path dependencies

These various initiatives highlight the burgeoning concept of holobiont public health within Finland's allergic disease landscape. Beneficial microbes are introduced as significant players in illness prevention and health promotion. New, microbially fortified, household products are available in the marketplace, kindergarten yards are being refurbished with natural elements, microbially enriched 'forest sandboxes' for children are placed in public playgrounds and recreational 'health forests' are established around Finland.[3] Although these initiatives remain on a small scale, they are sustained by the authoritative discursive reframing of allergy and associated conditions as results of 'nature deficiency' (Haahtela et al., 2024) and lack of adequate microbial contact.

However, as described above, these initiatives adopt markedly different approaches to facilitate microbial exposure. One approach leverages the market to encourage consumers to introduce 'good' microbes into their homes, while another engages in the 'microbial rewilding' (Mills et al., 2019) of urban environments to increase opportunities for public interaction with nature. In the former instance, microbes are incorporated into human habitats through various consumer products, while in the latter, human encounters with microbes are facilitated in natural settings inhabited by non-human organisms. This bifurcation reflects the multidisciplinary character of the ongoing research and development landscape, which combines biomedical and ecological expertise alongside a focus upon innovation.

I want to suggest that this bifurcation also reveals path dependencies inherent in public health practices. The proposed avenues of fostering microbial contact and generating associated health benefits exploit prevailing practices and echo prior public health strategies. One avenue is enriched consumer goods, which allow people to purchase health benefits at a premium. New material elements (microbes) and new meanings (their postulated health merits) are attached to established practices of personal healthcare and consumption. Innovative product development and marketing strategies promote a new class of health-enhancing products, comparable to probiotics and other functional foods, which carry scientifically validated health claims. Claims concerning the health benefits of microbial contact represent a 'market device' with which to steer consumer behaviour and secure competitive advantage for companies that have licensed the microbial extract, but similar market-based tactics are common also in public health (e.g. health labels). As this strategy suggests, individuals are conceptualised as consumers making choices based on their knowledge and values, and the task of public health is posited as one of educating people and encouraging informed decision-making that supports healthy lifestyles.

Another, more infrastructural strategy of promoting healthy microbial contact is the 'rewilding' of urban green spaces and built environments, such as kindergarten yards. Previous studies have highlighted urban green areas as facilitators of healthy lifestyle, such as physical activity, and proximity to these areas is associated with health benefits (Twohig-Bennett and Jones, 2018). Amid the present environmental poly-crisis, urban green spaces are also increasingly framed as sites for mitigating biodiversity loss and the effects of climate change, such as heatwaves and rainstorms (Tóth et al., 2015). Promoting salutary microbial contact through biodiverse flora and fauna is an additional incentive for the greening of urban spaces (Flies et al., 2018). Microbial rewilding multiplies opportunities for exposure by increasing the number and scope of green areas and making them more biodiverse through plant selection and by allowing decaying matter to stay on the ground. This approach, too, builds on pre-existing practices, such as commuting or walking, that take place outdoors. New elements and meanings are potentially attached to these practices, but this is not crucial for the performance of the practice in the same way as when purchasing a microbially enhanced product. In this strategy, opportunities for microbial contact are distributed in urban space, with the aim of exposing city dwellers to beneficial microbes during their everyday routines.

The two strategies are combined in the Nature Step to Health pilot programme described above, which addresses both individual health behaviours and the environments in which these behaviours unfold. The programme emphasises on the one hand lifestyle factors, particularly nutrition and physical activity, which are framed as matters of individual choice. On the other hand, it focuses on developing living environments conducive to nature connection and active mobility, which includes infrastructural aspects related to city planning and urban structure. On both dimensions, the joint objective is health and sustainability (Hämäläinen et al., 2023).

In these ways, the programme situates holobiont ideas within rather traditional health-promotion principles and practices, which centre on the individual and view the environment as presenting either opportunities or barriers to healthy behaviours (Patja et al., 2022). In effect, the new preventive paradigm is incorporated into a mainstream regime of non-communicable disease prevention characterised by a long-standing emphasis on lifestyle factors, such as diet and physical activity (Mayes, 2015). This framing undermines the ecosystemic perspective central to holobiont public health, as it fails to account for ecological relations, the totality of which determines health in each situation.

When positioned within this setting, health promoting microbial exposure is attached to established practices, such as consuming everyday goods and engaging in outdoor activities. Purchasing a microbially fortified bedsheet or allowing children to play in a biodiversity-rich kindergarten yard do not represent radically new microbial health practices, instead microbes are introduced into familiar practices with marginal change. Despite the promise, microbes are not foregrounded as dynamic non-humans materially shaping practices but remain in the background as supplements added to everyday consumer items or as invisible entities encountered in the environment. The general impression is thus one of sustained continuity rather than transformative shift both in the practices that are thought to promote everyday microbial contact and the policy strategies that govern these engagements.

Conclusion

In her recent book, Elizabeth Shove raises a pertinent question regarding whether 'new structures of knowing and doing, and new medical discourses [will] emerge around post-genomic theories, and how might such developments be guided, and perhaps limited, by dominant paradigms and by the institutions and practices associated with them?' (Shove, 2023: 22). This chapter has examined the biodiversity hypothesis, deeply rooted in microbiome science, and considered its potential as 'a new medical discourse' that has instigated 'new structures of knowing and doing' in the context of allergy prevention in Finland. Introducing the emergent paradigm of holobiont public health, I showed how relevant inventions within the allergy prevention realm are indeed 'guided, and perhaps limited, by dominant paradigms and by the institutions and practices associated with them' (Shove, 2023 41). More specifically, microbial allergy prevention is being attached to dominant practices of health promotion that emphasise individual choice and that frame the environment in relation to human activities.

While Latour (1988) highlighted microbes as a new class of transformative actants that through their associations changed society, other accounts of the 'bacteriological revolution' have stressed continuity and the persistence of existing practices (Worboys, 2000). When Pasteurian ideas about microbes emerged in the late 19th century, they encountered a set of established medical and healthcare practices. Microbes were incorporated into these practices, but rather than causing a comprehensive rupture this resulted in a set of smaller displacements that changed practices from within. For example, microbes gave a new rationale for existing practices of cleaning the environment and taking care of the body but did not engender radical change in daily life (Jauho, 2007).

It is not unreasonable to expect something similar in the case of microbiome science and holobiont public health. As this chapter has demonstrated, the biodiversity hypothesis has been introduced into illness prevention and health promotion against the backdrop of a complex set of practices that shape and constrain the integration of novel ideas and strategies into public health policy: 'attempts at steering or intervention do not occur in a vacuum. Existing policy, programmes and related activities already maintain or support extant practices and ways of life' (Maller, 2018: 131). In this constellation, the value of being exposed to microbes represents a concept that may subsequently modify existing practices from within. Because practice theory acknowledges this dynamic, it is a good analytical tool with which to assess the extent of change that innovations might usher in. Such analysis serves as a counterbalance to overly enthusiastic promissory narratives of revolutionary change, which are a typical feature of innovation discourse, including around microbiome science (Alivatos et al., 2015). While visions of more-than-human health are important and welcome, as they encourage a re-evaluation of our relationship with non-human others and a more balanced ecological co-existence, it is crucial to recognise the practices that condition the realisation of such projects. This calls for further studies of existing public health policies and strategies *as practices* in order to explore ways in which they might be adapted to better incorporate more-than-human models, such as holobiont public health.

Notes

1 See www.biwe.fi/en/home/. The group has gone through several iterations starting in 2015.
2 See www.biwe.fi/en/research/ and www.biwe.fi/en/nationwide-research-on-the-rewilding-of-kindergarten-yards-vahvistu/, for more details of the research.
3 https://healthforest.fi/ explains how forests heal people.

References

Aguirre, A.A., Ostfeld, R., Tabor, G., House, C. and Pearl, M. (eds.) (2022). *Conservation Medicine:* ***Ecological*** *health in practice*. Oxford: Oxford University Press.

Alivatos, A.P., Blaser, M., Brodie, E., Chun, M., Dangl, J., Donohue, T., Dorrestein, P., Gilbert, J., Green, J., Jansson, J., Knight, R., Maxon, M., McFall-Ngai, M., Miller, J., Pollard, K., Ruby, E., Taha, S. and Unified Microbiome Initiative Consortium (2015). 'A unified initiative to harness Earth's microbiomes: Transition from description to causality and engineering', *Science*, 350(6260): 507–508. https://doi.org/10.1126/science.aac8480.

Blaser, M.J. (2014). *Missing Microbes: How killing bacteria creates modern plagues.* London: Oneworld Publishing.

Blue, S., Shove, E., Carmona, C., and Kelly, M.P. (2016). 'Theories of practice and public health: understanding (un)healthy practices', *Critical Public Health*, 26(1): 36–50. https://doi.org/10.1080/09581596.2014.980396.

Blue, S., Shove, E. and Kelly, M.P. (2021). 'Obese societies: Reconceptualising the challenge for public health', *Sociology of Health and Illness*, 43(4): 1051–1067. https://doi.org/10.1111/1467-9566.13275.

Coutts, C., Forkink, A. and Weiner, J. (2014). 'The Portrayal of Natural Environment in the Evolution of the Ecological Public Health Paradigm', *International Journal of Environmental Research and Public Health*, 11(1): 1005–1019. https://doi.org/10.3390/ijerph110101005.

Flies, E.J., Skelly, C., Lovell, R., Breed, M. F., Phillips, D. and Weinstein, P. (2018). 'Cities, biodiversity and health: we need healthy urban microbiome initiatives', *Cities and Health*, 2(2): 143–150. https://doi.org/10.1080/23748834.2018.1546641.

Haahtela, T. (2019). 'A biodiversity hypothesis', *Allergy*, 74: 1445–1456. https://doi.org/10.1111/all.13763.

Haahtela, T., Bousquet, J. and Antó, J.M. (2024). 'From biodiversity to nature deficiency in human health and disease', *Porto Biomedical Journal*, 9(1), article 245. https://doi.org/10.1097/j.pbj.0000000000000245.

Haahtela, T., Laatikainen, T., Alenius, H., Auvinen, P., Fyhrquist N., Hanski, I., von Hertzen, L., Jousilahti, P., Kosunen, T., Markelova, O., Mäkelä, M., Pantelejev, V., Uhanov, M., Zilber, E. and Vartiainen, E. (2015). 'Hunt for the origin of allergy — comparing the Finnish and Russian Karelia', *Clinical and Experimental Allergy*, 45(5): 891–901. https://doi.org/10.1111/cea.12527.

Haahtela, T., Valovirta, E., Saarinen, K., Jantunen, J., Lindström, I., Kauppi, P., Laatikainen, T., Pelkonen, A., Saava, A., Tommila, E., Bousquet, J., Vasankari, T., Mäkelä, M. and the Allergy Program Group (2021). 'The Finnish Allergy Program 2008–2018: Society-wide proactive program for change of management to mitigate allergy burden', *Journal of Allergy and Clinical Immunology*, 148(2): 319–326. https://doi.org/10.1016/j.jaci.2021.03.037.

Halonen, J., Karvonen, A., Pasanen, T. and Samela, A. (2026). *Terveyattä luonnosta-ohjelma, 2026-2035.* Helsinki: Finnish Institute for Health and Welfare.

Hämäläinen, R-M., Halonen, J., Haveri, H., Prass, M., Virtanen, S., Salomaa, M-M., Sieppi, P. and Haahtela, T. (2023). 'Nature step to health 2022–2032: Interorganizational collaboration to prevent human disease, nature loss, and climate crisis', *The Journal of Climate Change and Health*, 10: 100194. https://doi.org/10.1016/j.joclim.2022.100194.

Hancock, T. (1993). 'Health, human development and the community ecosystem: three ecological models', *Health Promotion International*, 8(1): 41–47. https://doi.org/10.1093/heapro/8.1.41

Hanski, I., von Hertzen, L., Fyhrquist, N., Koskinen, K., Torppa, K., Laatikainen, T., Karisola, P., Auvinen, P., Paulin, L., Mäkelä, M., Vartiainen, T. Kosunen, T., Alenius, H. and Haahtela, T. (2012). 'Environmental biodiversity, human microbiota, and allergy are interrelated', *PNAS*, 109(21): 8334–8339. https://doi.org/10.1073/pnas.1205624109.

Hui, A., Schatzki, T. and Shove, E. (2017). *The Nexus of Practices: Connections, constellations, practitioners.* London: Routledge. https://doi.org/10.4324/9781315560816.

Hui, N., Grönroos, M., Roslund, M., Parajuri, A., Vari, H., Soinen, L., Laitinen, O., Sinkkonen, A. and the ADELE Research Group (2019) 'Diverse Environmental Microbiota as a Tool to Augment Biodiversity in Urban Landscaping Materials', *Frontiers of Microbiology*, 10, article 536. https://doi.org/10.3389/fmicb.2019.00536.

Jauho, M. (2007). *Kansanterveysongelman synty. Tuberkuloosi ja terveyden hallinta Suomessa ennen toista maailmansotaa.* Tutkijaliitto.

Landecker, H. (2016). 'Antibiotic Resistance and the Biology of History', *Body and Society*, 22(4): 19–52. https://doi.org/10.1177/1357034X14561341.

Latour, B. (1988). *The Pasteurization of France.* Cambridge, MA: Harvard University Press.

Latvala, J., von Hertzen, L., Lindholm, H. and Haahtela, T. (2005). 'Trends in prevalence of asthma and allergy in Finnish young men: a nationwide study from 1966 to 2003', *British Medical Journal*, 330(7501): 1186–1187. https://doi.org/10.1136/bmj.38448.603924.AE.

Lederberg, J. and McCray, A. T. (2001). 'Ome sweet 'omics: A genealogical treasury of words', *Scientist*, 15(7): 8.

Lerner, H. and Berg, C. (2017). 'A Comparison of three holistic approaches to health: One Health, EcoHealth, and Planetary Health', *Frontiers of Veterinary Science*, 4, article 163. https://doi.org/10.3389/fvets.2017.00163.

Lorimer, J. (2020). *The Probiotic Planet: Using life to manage life.* Minneapolis: University of Minnesota Press. https://doi.org/10.5749/j.ctv19cw9vg.

Mallee, H. (2017). 'The evolution of health as an ecological concept', *Current Opinion in Environmental Sustainability*, 25:28–32. https://doi.org/10.1016/j.cosust.2017.04.009.

Maller, C. (2015). 'Understanding health through social practices: performance and materiality in everyday life', *Sociology of Health and Illness*, 37(1): 52–66. https://doi.org/10.1111/1467-9566.12178.

Maller, C. (2018). *Healthy Urban Environments: More-than-human theories.* London: Routledge.

Mayes, C. (2015). *The Biopolitics of Lifestyle: Foucault, ethics and healthy choices.* London: Routledge.

McLeroy, K.R., Bibau, D., Steckler, A., and Glanz, K. (1988). 'An Ecological Perspective on Health Promotion Programs', *Health Education Quarterly*, 15(4): 351–377. https://doi/10.1177/109019818801500401.

Mills, J.G., Brookes, J., Gellie, N., Liddicoat, C., Lowe, A., Sydnor, H., Thomas, T., Weinstein, P. Weyrich, L., and Breed, M. (2019). 'Relating Urban Biodiversity to Human Health With the "Holobiont" Concept', *Frontiers of Microbiology*, 10, article 550. https://doi.org/10.3389/fmicb.2019.00550.

Parajuli, A., Grönroos, M., Siter, N., Puhakka, R., Vari, H., Roslund, M., Jumpponen, A., Nurminen, N., Laitinen, O., Hyöty, H., Rajaniemi, J. and Sinkkonen, A. (2018). 'Urbanization Reduces Transfer of Diverse Environmental Microbiota Indoors', *Frontiers of Microbiology*, 9, article 84. https://doi.org/10.3389/fmicb.2018.00084.

Patja, K., Absetz, P. and Rautava, P. (2022). *Terveyden edistäminen*. Duodecim.

Paxson, H. (2013). *The Life of Cheese: Crafting food and value in America.* Berkeley CA: University of California Press.

Platts-Mills, T.A.E. (2015). 'The Allergy Epidemics: 1870–2010', *Journal of Allergy and Clinical Immunology*, 136(1): 3–13. https://doi.org/10.1016/j.jaci.2015.03.048.

Puhakka, R., Rantala, O., Roslund, M. I., Rajaniemi, J., Laitinen, O. H., Sinkkonen, A and the Adele Research Group (2019). 'Greening of Daycare Yards with Biodiverse Materials Affords Well-Being, Play and Environmental Relationships', *International Journal of Environmental Research and Public Health*, 16(16), article 2948. https://doi.org/10.3390/ijerph16162948.

Raffaetà, R. (2023). *Metagenomic Futures: How microbiome research is reconfiguring health and what it means to be human*. London: Routledge.

Reckwitz, A. (2002). 'Toward a theory of social practices: a development in culturalist theorizing', *European Journal of Social Theory*, 5(2): 243–263. https://doi.org/10.1177/13684310222225432.

Rook, G.A.W., Adams, V., Hunt, J., Palmer, R., Martinelli, R. and Brunet, L.R. (2004) 'Mycobacteria and other environmental organisms as immunomodulators for immunoregulatory disorders', *Springer Seminars in Immunopathology* 25 (3–4): 237–255. https://doi.org/10.1007/s00281-003-0148-9.

Rosenberg, E. and Zilber-Rosenberg, I. (2013). *The Hologenome Concept: Human, animal, and plant microbiota*. London: Springer.

Roslund, M., Galitskya, P., Saarenpää, M. and Sinkkonen, A. (2024) 'Cultivar-dependent differences in plant bud microbiome and functional gene pathways in woody plants commonly used in urban green space', *Letters in Applied Microbiology*, 77(12), article ovae110. https://doi.org/10.1093/lambio/ovae110.

Roslund, M., Parajuli, A., Hui, N., Puhakka, R., Grönroos, M., Soininen, L., Nurminen, N., Oikarinen, S., Cinek, O., Kramná, L., Schroderus, A-M., Laitinen, O., Kinnunen, T., Hyöty, H., Sinkkonen, A., and the Adele research group (2022). 'A Placebo-controlled double-blinded test of the biodiversity hypothesis of immune-mediated diseases: Environmental microbial diversity elicits changes in cytokines and increase in T regulatory cells in young children', *Ecotoxicology and Environmental Safety*, 242, 113900. https://doi.org/10.1016/j.ecoenv.2022.113900.

Saarenpää, M., Roslund, M., Nurminen, N., Puhakka, R., Kummola, L., Laitinen, O., Hyöty, H. and Sinkkonen, A. (2024). 'Urban indoor gardening enhances immune regulation and diversifies skin microbiota: A placebo-controlled double-blinded intervention study', *Environment International*, 187, article 108705. https://doi.org/10.1016/j.envint.2024.108705.

Sariola, S. and Gilbert, S. (2020). 'Toward a Symbiotic Perspective on Public Health: Recognizing the Ambivalence of Microbes in the Anthropocene', *Microorganisms*, 8(5), article 746. https://doi.org/10.3390/microorganisms8050746.

Sender, R., Fuchs, S. and Milo, R. (2016). 'Are we really vastly outnumbered? Revisiting the ratio of bacterial to host cells in humans', *Cell*, 164(3): 337–340. https://doi.org/10.1016/j.cell.2016.01.013.

Shove, E. (2010) 'Beyond the ABC: climate change policy and theories of social change', *Environment and Planning A*, 42: 1273–1285. https://doi.org/10.1068/a42282.

Shove, E. (2023). *Connecting Practices: Large topics in society and social theory*. London: Routledge. https://doi.org/10.4324/9781003275107.

Shove, E., Pantzar, M. and Watson, M. (2012). *The Dynamics of Social Practice: Everyday life and how it changes*. London: Sage. https://doi.org/10.4135/9781446250655.

Shove, E. and Trentmann, F. (eds.) (2018). *Infrastructures in Practice: The dynamics of demand in networked societies*. London: Routledge. https://doi.org/10.4324/9781351106177.

Soininen, L., Roslund, M., Nurminen, N., Puhakka, R., Laitinen, O., Hyöty, H., Sinkkonen, A. and the Adele research group (2022). 'Indoor green wall affects health-associated commensal skin microbiota and enhances immune regulation: a randomized trial among urban office workers', *Scientific Reports*, 12: 6518. https://doi.org/10.1038/s41598-022-10432-4.

Soininen, L., Roslund, M., Tahvonen, O., Manninen, J., Hui, N., and Sinkkonen, A. (2024) 'Forestry- and agriculture-derived materials as bacterial supplements in immunomodulatory urban greening', *Urban Forestry and Urban Greening*, 101: 128492. https://doi.org/10.1016/j.ufug.2024.128492.

Strachan, D.P. (1989). 'Hay fever, hygiene, and household size', *British Medical Journal*, 299(6710): 1259–1260. https://doi.org/10.1136/bmj.299.6710.1259.

Strengers, Y. and Maller, C. (2018). 'Dynamic Non-humans in a Changing World', in Maller C. and Strengers, Y. (eds.) *Social Practices and Dynamic Non-Humans: Nature, materials and technologies*. London: Springer. 1–21. https://doi.org/10.1007/978-3-319-92189-1.

Tóth, A., Halajová, D. and Halaj, P. (2015). 'Green infrastructure: a strategic tool for climate change mitigation in urban environments', *Ecology and Safety*, 9: 132–138. www.scientific-publications.net/en/article/1000705/

Twohig-Bennett, C. and Jones, A. (2018). 'The health benefits of the great outdoors: A systematic review and meta-analysis of greenspace exposure and health outcomes', *Environmental research*, 166: 628–637. https://doi.org/10.1016/j.envres.2018.06.030.

Van Hul, M. and Cani, P.D. (2026). 'From microbiome to metabolism: Bridging a two-decade translational gap', *Cell Metabolism*, 38(1): 14–32. https://doi.org/10.1016/j.cmet.2025.10.011.

Velasquez-Manoff, M. (2012). *An Epidemic of Absence: A new way of understanding allergies and autoimmune diseases*. New York: Scribner.

von Hertzen L., Hanski, I. and Haahtela, T. (2011). 'Natural immunity. Biodiversity loss and inflammatory diseases are two global megatrends that might be related', *EMBO Reports*, 12: 1089–1093. https://doi.org/10.1038/embor.2011.195.

von Mutius, E., Fritzsch, C., Weiland, S., Röll, G., and Magnussen, H. (1992). 'Prevalence of asthma and allergic disorders among children in united Germany: a descriptive comparison', *British Medical Journal*, 305(6866): 1395–1399. https://doi.org/10.1136/bmj.305.6866.1395

Worboys, M. (2000). *Spreading Germs: Disease theories and medical practice in Britain, 1865–1900*. Cambridge: Cambridge University Press.

7

MICROBIAL ATMOSPHERES

Healthcare architectures as a 'more-than-human' dispositif

Nik Brown, Christina Buse, Daryl Martin and Sarah Nettleton

Introduction

This chapter focuses on three contrasting historical healthcare 'architectural dispositifs' (Yaneva, 2023; Martin et al. 2025), each designed with reference to changing conceptions of infectious disease, microbial transmission, care and prevention. We explore healthcare buildings as materially-discursive expressions of human-microbial co-evolution that, in turn, are continually reshaping traditions of architectural design. The term 'dispositif' describes how relationships to the microbial, as in the context of COVID-19, generate 'a physical mechanism and a heterogeneous ensemble consisting of architectural forms, spatial instructions, administrative measures, discourses, technologies and institutions' (Yaneva, 2022: 2).

More specifically, we examine the tensions inherent in architectural designs driven by the need to control, protect and manage human-microbial co-evolution particularly through the medium of the air, breath and breathing. Using three buildings, spanning a century from the 1910s, we reflect on the way atmospheric transmissibility prompts the re-configuring of common spatial typologies (Borch, 2008) generating the emergence of new forms of caring practice that hold within them trace memories of human-microbial pasts, whilst also presaging their as yet unknown futures. Here we are guided by Lefebvre's 'regressive-progressive' whereby 'the genesis of the present' can only be discerned by 'working our way back to the past and then retracing our steps' (1991: 65–66). In this way we treat healthcare architectures as historically overlapping assemblages which bring humans and microbes together in contrasting socio-material relationships.

DOI: 10.4324/9781003685210-9

We want to explore this theme, acknowledging the hitherto understated importance of breath as a prism through which to approach 'materialities of care' (Buse et al. 2018; Brown et al. 2020; Martin et al. 2025), and the ways in which breath is implicated in the temporal and spatial ordering and experience of illness (Oxley and Russell, 2020). Respiratory infectivity renders the act of breathing as something to be explicated (Irigaray, 1999), planned, and cared for (Macnaughton, 2020). As a medium of transmission, air becomes explicit (Sloterdijk, 2009), 'part of an air-conditioning system that makes our life possible' (Latour, 2004). Breathing is institutionalised and encoded in cultural rules (Lande, 2007) and is particularly so for the 'coughing body' (Brown et al., 2021b). The built environment becomes a key point of tension when exposure to microbial threat occurs in aerobiologically fluid encounters between bodies within particular buildings (Garnett, 2020), and especially hospitals (Brown et al. 2020, 2021a, 2021b).

To design the air is a matter of struggling to remember the forgettable and envision the invisible. 'Always there', Irigaray (1999) writes, the air 'allows itself to be forgotten'. Instead, an aerographic perspective prompts us to 'begin with' (Jackson and Fannin, 2011) and 'take to' (Connor, 2006) the air. Opening the window on air prompts us to ask questions differently and overturn the 'oblivion' of the air (Rousell and Lupton, 2025). The air is clouded in doubt, and hospitals can often be seen as environments of aerographic uncertainty where air's movement becomes an epistemic problem of un/knowability.

Air, Connor writes, fragments the borders of bodies and buildings, rendering space as 'produced and dynamic, rather than absolute and given' (2006: 121). Buildings lend bodies metaphorical sturdiness while bodies give buildings their liveliness. 'This contrast is at its most intense', Connor suggests, '… when the physical processes in question are least material … those carried on or in the air' (Connor, 2006: 118). Air's disassembling of the building is possibly nowhere more apparent than in the world of the microbial. Much of the recent 'turn' towards aerography is attributed to 'an increasingly visible breaking down of air' (Nieuwenhuis, 2016).

Our three architectural dispositifs correspond to the periods before and since the introduction of antibiotics in the 1950s and allow us to reflect on questions of architectural design in the context of antimicrobial resistance (AMR). Our first architectural dispositif, from the 'pre-antibiotic era', focuses on the Papworth tuberculosis village just outside Cambridge in the UK, established in 1917. Here we explore the design and use of outdoor huts housing patients in continuous open-air 'aerotherapeutic' conditions. Our second dispositif, from the antibiotic era, is a 'modern' multistorey hospital that opened in the late 1970s in a provincial northern British city. The hospital can be understood as a classic of its type, built with economies of scale, efficiency and budget at the forefront of the design rationale. And our final dispositif is an infectious diseases hospital explicitly built with an architectural brief for the 'post-antibiotic future'. The result is a strikingly innovative architecture, but one which is also riven with complex and difficult aero-material tensions. In each of these discussions we draw on archival historical and secondary sources, interviews (with patients, carers and hospital staff), hospital site visits, ethnographic observations and walking interviews. Ethics approval was granted through the UK NHS and our University social science ethics board. Many of these methodological elements are discussed in greater depth elsewhere (Brown et al., 2021a and 2021b; Martin et al., 2025).

The papworth TB settlement: A pre-antibiotic dispositif

The dispositif we focus on here is centred on the architectural relationship to the tubercle bacillus organism at the end of the nineteenth century and the opening decades of the twentieth. Our chosen architecture is a small-scale model of a rectangular outdoor wooden hut carefully handcrafted by its resident occupant, a patient at the Papworth tuberculosis 'colony' during the 1930s. The model is roughly the size of a large shoebox and forms part of London's Science Museum Wellcome Trust exhibition. To the front, the visitor can peer through two half doors into a cosy interior simply furnished with a single bed covered in a neat little pink woollen blanket and pillow. The hut has top-hinged panel openings at the sides and back allowing for cross-ventilation and the free movement of air. The roof is a gently sloping conical shape tapered on four sides, on top of which sits a ventilation chimney fitted with open wooden louvre slats. The accompanying text explains that 'The open and airy design was seen as the most effective way to treat the disease' in the period before antibiotics. A nearby photograph shows a long row of the huts disappearing into the distance, set against a tree-lined backdrop with residents in the foreground.

Prior (1988, 1992) traces the way miasmic theories of contagion became architecturally embedded in the classic 'fresh air wards' of the nineteenth century (see also Adams, 2008; Drake, 1997). This is a humoral medical discourse in which maladies become matters of atmospheric aetiology arising from zymotic gaseous chemical processes and mephitic fermentation. Resulting vapours and stagnating fumes must be dispersed to prevent sickness. Torpid air must not be allowed to become motionless and fester. It must move, circulate and refresh. The resulting architectural expression of miasmic discourse is the sanatoria and the 'pavilion' (Forty, 2003; Kisacky, 2005), etymologically from papillon (French), the butterfly tent. The hospital pavilion inverts internal and external space, detached from the main building, often having a radial tent-like cylindrical shape with no stagnant dark corners. The pavilion also uniformly distances patients one from another, the flow of air and light separating the bodies of the sick, and the bodies of buildings, into neatly divided atmospheres. The pavilion ward 'spatially isolated everything from everything by oceans of fresh natural air' (Kisacky, 2005). Wards would commonly be heated by a central stove, drawing air in towards the chimney to be evacuated at the apex of a vaulted roof. Beds would be wheeled outside to surrounding verandas, balconies and gardens for convalescence and 'air bathing' (Gauvain, 1933; Hobday and Dancer, 2013). The classic Nightingale ward would be south-facing and glazed floor-to-ceiling. Well into the mid-twentieth century, building designs for the sunlit 'fresh air cure' were the mainstay of tuberculosis treatment in the pre-antibiotic 'age' or 'era' (Blundell Jones, 2016: 267).

The huts at Papworth seemed to have varied somewhat but were modelled on the classic wooden cabin where TB 'colonists' would be accommodated for anywhere between several months and even years in some cases. As Bryder (1984) notes in a broader history of the Papworth sanatorium endeavour:

> Actual treatment at Papworth was based first and foremost on fresh air, or 'aerotherapy' as it was sometimes known. On arrival, patients were admitted to the hospital section for examination, but were generally quickly transferred to the sanatorium section, which consisted of open-air shelters.
>
> *(Bryder, 1984: 377)*

Papworth was founded in 1917 by Pendrill Varrier-Jones who would go on to become a leading tuberculosis treatment pioneer establishing this distinctly social-utopian 'village settlement' where patients were housed, often with their families, in bespoke buildings and structures. Varrier-Jones oversaw the expansion of the village to include huts, cottages, workshops and leisure facilities. The focus at Papworth centred on the environment of the body, rather than targeting the internal causes of disease. The approach was modelled on an idealised romantic garden village imaginary, reflecting the deeper late-Victorian reactions to industrial society. This may account for the bucolic-tinted praise the colony would routinely receive in the press with *The Times* feting the settlement as '... the most successful socio-medical experiment of our times... a proved method of the treatment of the tuberculous ... A Utopian dream... a living example of the success of high ideals, realised in practice' (*The Times,* 8th July 1927: 11).

One press piece, describing the 'Happiest village on earth', notes how 'victims of the "white scourge" pass through probationary stages' ... onto 'the "colony" of one-man bungalows grouped around a common 'mess hall, where he sleeps in fresh air' (*Daily Mail*, 5th July 1926: 7). Outdoor dwelling and exposure to the English weather, Varrier-Jones believed, had a stimulating metabolic effect on the immune system suppressing infection, and making necessary '... a complete return to Nature, and explicit obedience to Nature's laws as possible' (Varrier-Jones, 1916).

Bryder's wider historical account of TB colonies touches very briefly on huts and draws on several archival sources noting that one patient (Durham) recalled being allocated a hut and living two 'happy years' there, 'free as a bird, with the wind coming through four canvas flaps on the hut sides, with all the scents of the countryside flowing in – some good, some bad.' (Bryder, 1984: 377). Another patient remembered waking up to find their boots frozen solid to the floor, claiming that this was not unusual. In an interview, one of the nurses remembered that false teeth would often be found icebound in a bedside glass. Patients were however generously 'supplied with a waterproof blanket to keep the snow off their beds' (Bryder, 1984: 377).

Varrier-Jones paid careful personal attention to the architectural design of the dwellings on the estate, insisting that 'the windows of Papworth are always open, so that no concentration of bacilli can occur to infect anyone' (Varrier-Jones, 1930: 268). He would take the trouble to sketch the layout of huts and cottage dwellings, the situation of balconies, and the use of glazing to maximise light. Cottages would be, Bryder notes, 'semi-detached, two storeyed, with three bedrooms, and a veranda on the first floor for the tuberculous patient. Windows were to be permanently open'. (Bryder, 1984: 380). As with the huts, an emphasis was placed on the open porosity of buildings and a more seamless relationship between internal and external spaces.

Papworth had, certainly by the late 1920s, established a commercially viable market in the manufacture and sale of outdoor structures for the tuberculous patient, offered to hospitals, domestic homes and local authorities. Writing in 1907, Hall notes that '... much is heard... of the chalet type, or wood hut for a single patient, and its trifling cost as compared with a permanent sanatorium' (Hall, 1907: 138). *The Nottingham Evening Post* also describes a pragmatic solution to 'fresh air' dwelling:

> treatment for tubercular disease can be provided ... without great expense. ... Many local authorities now encourage the use of the backyard for the purpose of open-air treatment, and in Bermondsey the Borough Council even lends poor consumptives wooden huts so that they may go to bed in the garden, and so get almost as much good as they would if accommodated in a sanatorium... Shelters should be rectangular in order to afford protection on two adjoining sides, whichever way the wind blows, while being open on the other two sides.
>
> *(Nottingham Evening Post, August 6th 1912: 3)*

Campbell (2005) suggests that from the mid nineteenth to twentieth centuries, tuberculosis had become a lightning rod for progressive architectural forces spanning clinical hygienist modernism, the Bauhaus, the Garden City (England) and Life Reform (Germany) movements, focusing on light, air and sun. Campbell also pays attention to a lively early twentieth century market in the revolving summer house, installed in the grounds of sanatoria including City Hospital in Edinburgh:

> Unlike the other modernist architectural features… the summer house retained a vernacular Arts and Crafts appearance that belied its fashionable, therapeutic role. It was the inexpensive flat-pack shelter with no historicist pretensions that pointed the way to late twentieth-century DIY, home-assembly, prefabricated units that range from furniture to garden sheds.
> *(Campbell, 2005: 481)*

Today, the legacy of Papworth's huts endures with one of the streets named 'Hut Field Lane'. A full-size replica TB hut stands in the grounds of the now state-of-the-art hospital, 'a permanent reminder of our origins as a colony for tuberculosis patients… our past, now sits proudly beside our futuristic present building' (Papworth NHS Foundation Trust, 2023). In the cultural memory surrounding the Papworth settlement, the hut remains an enduring iconic architectural motif signifying the world before antibiotics.

The Seacole Hospital – an 'antibiotic dispositif'

The exemplar dispositif we want to focus on in the context of the 'antibiotic age' is a classic mid-1970s-built hospital located in a provincial northern British city. When first built, Seacole (pseudonym) was described as an example of a highly economical design. A detailed building study in 1977 noted the intention to reduce the 'huge bulk of the building and to create a domestic scale to which a human could relate' and 'to maximise the number of beds … to ease nursing care'. Crucially, the brief was 'to design a very cheap hospital within stringent … cost limits.' (*The Architect's Journal*, 1977: 1021).

The Seacole hospital estate comprised four tower blocks each having an internal courtyard allowing it to be naturally lit from sliding glazed windows wrapping continuously around the outside of the building. The towers are connected by an enclosed 'hospital street' or corridor, measuring nearly three hundred metres in length but only just over four metres wide, through which passes almost all of the hospital's flow in patients, clinicians, visitors, equipment, laundry and supplies. Today, clinical staff are conscious of the infection transmission risks presented by the 'street' and talk of 'getting by' and 'making do' in a high-density low-budget building.

Medical architectural historians (Bud, 2007) have written about how the advent of antibiotics in the mid-20th century catalysed a profound reconfiguration of healthcare delivery – not merely in terms of therapeutic protocols, but also in the spatial logics of medicine. The newfound ability to treat infections pharmacologically rather than through environmental and atmospheric management, allowed for the concentrated densification and increased patient turnover within the tight geometries of more Fordist hospital architectures.

As Chandler (2019) argues, antibiotics became 'infrastructurally' constitutive of wider elements in a socio-technical system absorbed into everyday life and clinical environments to the extent that atmospheres, including the physical architectural design of aero-helio-therapeutic approaches – were displaced by pharmacology. In short, antibiotics signalled a 'dramatic break' from the tradition of sanatoria design (Adams et al., 2016), turning 'away from Nightingale's principles, closing their windows and shutting out the sun' (Swain, 2013: 35).

Of course, this transformation cannot be attributed solely to antibiotics: it co-evolves with other forces at work. The oil crisis of the 1970s, coupled with tightening public budgets, reinforced architectural moves towards energy conservation and spatial compactness. Openable windows and the external environment itself were now seen to threaten the fragile technology-dependent integrity of high-rise, deep-density buildings that we have come to associate with modern healthcare environments. The hermetically sealed hospital atmosphere has become a matter of centrally-controlled 'air management' (Latour, 2004). Many contemporary hospitals can be said to have increasingly become a sealed biome, dependent on mechanical air management systems creating a new kind of medical ecology, mediated not by sunlight or fresh air but by HVAC (heating, ventilation and air conditioning) systems, antibacterial surfaces and pharmaceutical routines. The hospital's therapeutic efficacy now hinged on producing what might be termed a post-environmental clinical space.

Antibiotics arguably supported the questionable impression that an aerotherapeutic attention to space was no longer needed but as early as the 1960s a piece in *The Architect's Journal* critically reflects on the '... increase in turn-over of patients... overcrowding ... The failure of antibiotics to solve the general problem of hospital infection has ... stimulated a re-examination of hospital design... [and] ventilation' (Sommerville, 1960: 9). Kisacky (2017) expands on this theme, arguing that the 'design freedom [from the need for fresh air] was short-lived. ... antibiotic treatment of nosocomial infections was followed by a resurgence of ... antibiotic-resistant strains ... so high that a number of hospital administrators considered shutting down their facilities rather than continuing to produce hospital-acquired infections' (Kisacky, 2017: 341).

Illustrating many of these features, our study focused on the question of AMR in the context of healthcare delivery for cystic fibrosis (CF) patients in a number of contemporary hospitals including Seacole, each typical of 'antibiotic hospital architectures' from the latter half of the twentieth century. Our research set out to map the real-world pathways, journeys and flows of bodies and bodies of air through clinical space.

Until the 1990s, people with CF would routinely meet in open hospital wards, adjoining games rooms, waiting areas and on residential holidays. This interactional intimacy changed fundamentally with the identification of resistant bacteria traced to cross-infection through interpersonal contact (Conway, 2008). Living with CF has increasingly come to depend upon a hygienic regime of atmospheric segregation, ritualised etiquettes of social distancing and a keen acuity to infection risks carried on the air. The body of the CF patient has been transfigured into a vaporous source of infectious transmissibility to be isolated, imposing new self-pedagogies of hygienic prudence (Brown, et al. 2021a; Lowton and Gabe, 2006) and containment within 'circuits of hygiene' (Fox, 1997; see also the idea of 'sterility as a product of spatial ordering' (Mesman, 2009: 1705)).

When the Seacole Hospital was first built it was possible to fully open its wrap-around sliding aluminium windows, allowing for generous cross-ventilation as a means of reducing airborne hospital infections. However, safety legislation has since required window openings in public buildings to be restricted to 10 centimetres. Interviews with colleagues responsible for the hospital estate described how this radically reduced airflow, focusing concerns on airborne transmission and resulting in an uncomfortably warm atmosphere, increasing the need for mechanical ventilation. Harry, a building manager at Seacole, described how air quality had remained an intractable problem until the arrival of a new colleague, Adam, who had transferred from a nearby Victorian-built hospital. Adam and Harry described how the older hospital had inspired them to imagine ways of increasing natural ventilation.

After some trial and error, they designed discrete aluminium horizontal bars to be retro-fitted to the hospital's windows, allowing restrictors to be removed and the windows to be fully openable once again. Both Harry and Adam spoke nostalgically of the old Victorian era hospital, its vaulted ceilings, full-height windows, its spaciousness compared to the more compact 1970s modern estate. They discussed the old hospital's fixtures and fittings, and the use of copper, credited with natural antibacterial properties.

Much of our fieldwork centred on these historical tensions between competing air regimes, especially the ways in which windows come into conflict with air conditioning and heating systems. Cooper (2002) has written about how concepts of 'healthy air' change over time. For example, the 1900s campaigns extolling the benefits of external fresh air gave way in the twentieth century to industry-driven advertising promoting the modern advantages of air-conditioning for productivity and workplace output. Air 'conditioning' and 'air management' came to promise the conditioning of managed bodies in schools, hospitals and especially in offices and factories. Windows became contested ground between managerial and subordinate subjects. Following from our discussion above, in a walking interview, Harry shows us the original air ventilation system built into the fabric of the hospital back in the 1970s. But in his 20 years at the hospital, he has never known the system to be operated and nobody is sure anymore where the 'master switch' actually is. It's simply more obvious to open a window, he suggests.

Uncertainties about the air and its qualities were widely shared. In our research, medical staff and patients spoke of their anxieties about the air but were unsure whether and for how long bacteria 'linger in the air'. Changing the air, the rate of exchange, and its implications for infections in the air is, in most respects, a matter of guesswork. Envisioning aerographic risk is a question of having to speculatively 'imagine the atmosphere' but without really knowing (Wagenfeld, 2008). As one CF practitioner put it to us, the atmosphere of a room is an acute source of doubt:

> how much you mitigate it by opening a window? I don't know whether there is less risk [in] big open spaces, and the air exchange is different, I'm not sure ... all the infections that we see largely is airborne, and I don't know ... having wipeable surfaces is a benefit, but does it reduce airborne transmission? I don't know. I doubt it ... the one thing I really worry about ... is when a patient's been in the same area for a few hours ... I just imagine the atmosphere in that room full of bacteria ... and then the next person goes in ... So, we normally just ... open all the windows.
>
> *(Rachel, physiotherapist, Seacole)*

For people at risk of cross-infection, the air is imagined hydrologically as having a certain unruly leakiness, becoming an indeterminate source of liquid defilement and disorder. The fluid translucency of the air renders the atmosphere unclassifiable, neither one thing nor another. Always given to turbulence, clinical air is in a constant state of flux, threatening the orderliness of spatial boundaries and classificatory schema.

There are innumerable moments when uncertain questions of atmospheric transmission arise in the everyday life of the respiratory clinic, especially when patients are asked to provide sputum samples for microbiology diagnosis or to 'clear' their airways. This can include the administration of nebulised hypertonic saline inhaled to saturate the lungs before 'coughing up'. Specialist CF physiotherapists will usually be responsible for managing sputum sampling, assisting patients to 'produce' fluid from the lungs using direct physical contact:

> Some [rooms] have windows ... the Friday physio room doesn't ... I'll open the windows, if I've been getting people coughing and clearing stuff or have

> done a nebuliser … try and get the air flow through the room before I bring someone else in … often … you don't really have a lot of time to let any air flow through before you get someone else in (Mandy, physiotherapist).

One estates manager at Seacole guided us onto the roof of the hospital and pointed to an immense atmospheric plant machinery on the rooftop above. There's very little roof space left to be able to accommodate further air handling, plus it can't be retrofitted to such a compact building with few ceiling voids. For clinical staff in respiratory care, negative air is therefore largely an atmospheric aspiration, especially in the treatment of CF outpatients. A CF nurse at Seacole puts it, '… ideally we would need the negative pressure rooms… all we can do … is open the windows to get some fresh air … by no way perfect. They [windows] don't open very far, but yeah, they do open. So opening a window and trying to keep the door open for that half an hour, but logistically it can be quite difficult'.

A hospital-based microbiologist wasn't convinced of the evidence for negative pressure rooms. Highly dangerous pathogens like resistant non-tuberculous Mycobacteria and Mycobacterium abscessus may have multiple routes of environmental transmission beyond the temporarily purified world of a controlled pressure atmosphere. The 'evidence that it [air pressure management] will make a difference', he says, 'isn't really there … it massively adds complexity … and cost'. He went on to talk about Victorian buildings, fresh air wards, balconies, windows and the 'rate of air change'.

Again, the increased awareness of the dependence of life on competing air technics is suggestive of Sloterdijk's 'airquakes' (2004: 89), the life-threatening collision of atmospheres, in which 'to breathe' can no longer be simply assumed but must be technically accomplished. Air becomes vulnerable to mechanical, electrical and budget failure. Latour reflects on the technically mediated nature of air 'conditioning' writing: '… You are on life support, it's fragile, it's technical, it's public, it's political, it could break down – it is breaking down – it's being fixed, you are not too confident of those who fix it' (Latour, 2004: 3). In an airquake, economically complex architectural systems are given to self-defeating contradiction. The densification and concentration of the healthcare environment comes with unintended atmospheric costs. Whilst Sloterdijk tends to reflect on historically dramatic moments of life-threatening violence and subjugation, many such quakes are instead architecturally far more mundane and routine (Borch, 2008). It is this unobservability that makes it possible for the hidden design politics of atmospheric control to go unquestioned.

Malmo IDU – a post-antibiotic dispositiff

Our final architectural dispositif is a building specifically designed to deliver a hospital for a 'post-antibiotic' future, shaped around the SARS outbreaks some years earlier, the worsening AMR crisis (especially in tuberculosis), but also haemorrhagic infections (Ebola), and a pandemic imaginary anticipating the COVID-19 emergency yet to come. The establishment of the Skåne hospital reads across the past, present and the future in socio-materially reflecting on the kinds of architectures adapted to life lived with the prospect of pandemic infectious disease (Yaneva, 2022). Skåne's University Hospital's Infectious Diseases Unit (IDU) constructed between 2008–2010, is located in the Swedish city of Malmo and was designed by C.F. Møller together with Malmo's LINK Arkitektur. The resulting building is an iconic spherical landmark in the city. Here we retrace the history of hospital's design, drawing on interviews, site visits, walking interviews with hospital staff, and secondary sources.

Consciously reflecting the rotunda pavilion design, the building is arranged over six levels in a circular hollow disc. Two of the hospital's doctors recall the importance in their early planning of the need to give 'consideration of healthcare architecture design precedents from the pre-antibiotic era that might be relevant in the post-antibiotic era' (Holmdahl and Lanbeck, 2013: 35). Inpatient isolation rooms occupy the outer ring of three levels facing towards the immediate neighbourhood. The outer layer is specifically reserved for patients, their visitors and the removal of waste via dedicated lifts. Clinical and administrative services are housed in the inner ring facing towards a central courtyard and hospital entrance. Each of the patient levels has seventeen individual isolation rooms which can be entered through doors from an exterior wrap-around partially glazed balcony walkway, or alternatively through doors from the inner clinical ring.

The hospital is therefore architecturally bisected between purity and impurity (Douglas, 1966), with an inner 'clean' 'circuit of hygiene' (Fox, 1997: 649) dedicated to clinicians and ancillary staff, and an outer 'contaminated' circuit reserved for those carrying infections or visitors. There is a sense that providing external entry points into each isolation room keeps the patient 'outside' and distanced from the inner workings of the hospital. The whole architecture is carefully zoned through a series of spaces that can be closed off and partitioned, minimising the risk of cross-infection and representing control through 'segregated design' (Yaneva, 2022) years in advance of COVID-19.

The entire top floor of the hospital is a giant air ventilation and filtration plant. Two of the hospital's clinicians involved in its conception and design note that IDUs have '... traditionally have been located as freestanding facilities on the outskirts of... hospital grounds'. Instead, they set out to bring infectious disease into close proximity with the rest of the hospital adopting '... technical solutions like separate and advanced ventilation, isolated elevators, separate sewage systems, and exterior entrances to patient rooms (and outdoor air) via circulation balconies... [separating] the flow or circulation of patients with contagious diseases from other patients'. Their guiding rationale for the design of the hospital hinged on three principles of 'Far Away Yet Nearby, Flexibility, and Defined Links' (Holmdahl and Lanbeck, 2013: 35–36).

For Yaneva (2022), COVID-19 made ventilation a primary concern in architecture recalling pre-antibiotic glazing and airflow design preferences (Prior, 1988). The Malmo Unit's outer deck or balcony is encircled with full length glazed panels offset to each other and allowing for continual ventilation and unobstructed views of the city, keeping the patient 'outside' and yet sheltered from exposure to wind and rain. However, '... too much enclosure or shelter on the exterior paths' they note '... could violate the principle that fresh outdoor air reduces infection transmission risk' (Holmdahl and Lanbeck, 2013: 35) and resemble a sealed corridor, not unlike the hospital street at Seacole discussed above.

For the lead architect, this use of glass panelling was a design decision aimed at creating a particular architectural affect, allowing openness as well as protection. The glass frontage positions the building within a long-standing tradition shaped by principles of 'Licht, Luft und Öffnung' – or, light, air and openness. The architect explained that this attention had been formulated in relation to environmental evidence-based medicine 'working side by side' with the architectural brief to take sympathetic account of lengthy patient stays. During this time, isolated patients would need, he suggested, as much access to outside views as possible, whilst also delivering a degree of segregated sterility. He stressed the importance of a 'clear view from the bed', echoing principles of modernist sanatoria design like that of Alvar Aalto's intention that healthcare architecture function as a medical instrument. Colomina suggests these architectural spaces shifted from a concern with the vertical person to a focus on the horizontally inclined 'figure stretching always towards the light of the sun' (Colomina, 2019: 67).

Each isolation room has two anterooms, with heavy air-sealed doors, one leading outside, and one to the inner clinical area. Strict protocols determine which doors can be opened and which should be closed, regulating air exchanges. Anterooms offer a striking parallel example to the architecturally defensive typologies discussed by Christian Borch in his elaboration of Sloterdijk's foam architectures (Borch, 2008). In effect, anterooms work to defend the internal bedroom from outside risks through securitised, semi-public spaces that act as 'a psycho-social immune system that can regulate the degree to which it is sealed off from the outside world as it requires' (Sloterdijk, 2004: 578).

For clinicians, anterooms and individual entrances recalled the pre-antibiotic era department that had existed on the site previously. The anteroom would create an air barrier while maintaining optimal flow and control (Holmdahl and Lanbeck, 2013). Le Corbusier, in The Radiant

City (Le Corbusier, 1967), anticipates this conditioning of the air, equating the 'genuine goals of architecture' with 'the need to provide exact air' (Le Corbusier, 1967: 40) giving 'the lung the constant which is the prerequisite of its functioning' (Le Corbusier, 1967: 42). Likewise, the protected character of the anteroom connects with Sloterdijk's analysis of apartment design in the 20th century.

However, like our discussion of windows at Seacole above, doors also have their politics. During site visits, we found that nursing staff often struggle to open airtight doors made even heavier by negative air pressure. A hospital manager took us aside and explained how anteroom doors from the bedrooms to the external balcony would often be found propped open with chairs or other bedroom furnishings. Echoing themes from our first dispositif above, the patients, he explained, like to listen to the noise of the city and breathe the outside air rather than inside air. In so doing patients and their visitors subvert highly sensitive air purification and pressure systems. These and other unintended adaptations to the original architectural designs of the building are a common feature as buildings transition from conception to use. For example, the patient rooms were all designed with single-occupancy 'isolation' in mind but within only a few years of use, many individual rooms had been given over to multiple patient occupancy to deal with the shortage of beds. Buildings designed to partition the airs of individual patients can be open to adaptive interpretative flexibility with the intentions of designers continually open to revision by building users (Gieryn, 2002).

As has been argued with respect to this building, even lab-like architectures of atmospheric separation can be highly porous and leaky. In this case it has proved quite problematic to depend on the strict separation of the building's contaminated outer perimeter, and the clean inner ring occupied by staff. Beyond the segregated airs of the IDU, visitors and staff will travel together on Malmo's transport system. It can be difficult to completely maintain that pure threshold between these outer and inner worlds. Calvillo's argument that the use of buildings will always be provisional, and indeed should be considered experimental, is persuasive (Calvillo, 2018). Calvillo follows Sloterdijk on the use of air to understand questions of design but rejects his 'metaphorical reading of architecture as enclosure'. Instead, Calvillo argues that we should consider architecture 'not simply as creating envelopes for climate control, but as involving the actual design of atmospheres where the air is not only a conditioner of well-being but also a material for the construction of certain modes of sociality' (Calvillo, 2018: 44). The dispositif of containment (Yaneva, 2022) is always contingent, never completely determined by design, echoing Calvillo's suggestion that we 'reduce the expectations of architecture and shift from constructing the social to facilitating socialities' instead (Calvillo, 2018: 42).

Concluding discussion

In the context of AMR and COVID-19, air is possibly undergoing a renaissance in the interplay of historical memory and impending dystopian doom. 'Perhaps we can prepare for the looming post-antibiotic era' writes Swain, 'by taking some lessons from the pre-antibiotic age...' (Swain, 2013: 34). Kembel et al. (2014) point to the relatively ignored inter-connectedness of architectural design and microbial ecology and note the nascent interest in buildings in which humans spend the majority of their time as 'multi-species ecosystems'.

In an article that speculates on 'infection control in the post-antibiotic era', Dancer (2013) champions a return to air, and in both popular and expert biological discourse, hospitals and domestic environments are being re-imagined as bodies having their own microbiome (Adams et al., 2016). Like skin and lungs, indoor cavities and surfaces have become a refuge for antibiotically resistomes. First AMR and now COVID-19 have given rise to a new biopolitical opening with which to 'rethink' the implications of a culture of enclosed sterility that has dominated the design of the hospital environment throughout much of the twentieth century and into the present.

It is now possible to see that in parallel with the aerographic turn in social theory, there is a growing interest in microbiology on external 'fresh' air as a source of atmospheric 're-wilding', the de-domestication of the otherwise lifeless air of the internal environment. Windowless air-conditioned hospitals, it is argued, are over-populated with harmful pathogens, compromising the healthy biodiversity of building ecology and allowing resistance to flourish uncontested. Microbiologists have shown that ventilation rates in old hospitals with passive air flow have been found to be far greater than in newer hospitals with engineered ventilation, such that we're coming 'full circle in hospital design' (Escombe et al., 2007: 68). Large naturally ventilated hospital spaces, once windows are closed, have been seen to quadruple infection risks (Noakes et al., 2012).

As we suggest above, air is even becoming enfolded in a material discourse of atmospheric 'rewilding' not dissimilar to that happening in the context of probiotic micro-fauna (intestinal worms for the treatment of autoimmune bowel disease) and the hotly debated re-introduction of charismatic megafauna (see Lorimer, 2020). Going probiotic meshes with mounting concerns around the bio-depletion of both the body and the natural environment, reflected in attempts to somehow reverse the logics of sterile purity through restorative bio-diversifying interventions. The rigid boundaries of the built environment are in this way being called into question.

In tracing the trajectory of these three historical architectural dispositifs, healthcare buildings can be seen to serve as materially discursive expressions of human-microbial co-evolution, continuously reshaped by shifting socio-material paradigms of infection and care. From the aerotherapeutic focus of the pre-antibiotic era to the densified, hermetically sealed post-environmental clinical spaces of the antibiotic age, architectural design has struggled to account for the 'invisible' and 'forgettable' medium of air. Today, the dual pandemic crises of AMR and SARS-CoV invite a return to questions of ventilation and the re-conceptualisation of the built environment as multi-species ecosystems rather than sites of sterile enclosure. Post-antibiotic imaginaries of atmospheric re-wilding challenge the twentieth-century logic of total isolation. How spaces are practiced, inhabited and even subverted in unfolding processes of use underscores the ongoing provisionality and contingency of architectural design intent. Many of our themes here echo Blue and Spurling's (2017) analysis of hospitals demonstrating how infrastructures operate not merely as technical supports but as integral elements in the coordination and reproduction of interdependent practices of care, administration, and movement. By moving away from understandings of buildings as solidly fixed envelopes towards the design of atmospheres that facilitate aerographic sociality, healthcare architecture can potentially be made more open to a future of evolving aerographic design. It may therefore become possible to rethink the architectures of the built environment more porously through concepts of breath, breathing and respiratory relationality.

References

Adams, A. (2008). *Medicine by Design: The architect and the modern hospital, 1893-1943*. Minneapolis: University of Minnesota Press.

Adams, R.I., Bhangar, S., Dannemiller, K.C., Eisen, J.A., Fierer, N., Gibert, J. Green, J., Marr, L., Miller, S., Siegel, J., Stephens, B., Waring, M. and Bibby, K. (2016). 'Ten questions concerning the microbiomes of buildings', *Building and Environment*, 109: 224–234. http://dx.doi.org/10.1016/j.buildenv.2016.09.001.

Blue, S. and Spurling, N. (2017). 'Qualities of connective tissue in hospital life: how complexes of practices change' in Hui, A., Schatzki, T. and Shove, E. (eds.) *The Nexus of Practices: Connections, constellations, practitioners*. London: Routledge. 24–37. https://doi.org/10.4324/9781315560816.

Blundell Jones, P. (2016). *Architecture and Ritual: How buildings shape society*. London: Bloomsbury Publishing.

Borch, C. (2008). 'Foam architecture: Managing co-isolated associations', *Economy and Society*, 37(4): 548–571. https://doi.org/10.1080/03085140802357943.

Brown, N., Buse, C., Lewis, A., Martin, D. and Nettleton, S. (2020.) 'Air care: An "aerography" of breath, buildings and bugs in the cystic fibrosis clinic', *Sociology of Health and Illness*, 42(5): 972–986. https://doi.org/10.1111/1467-9566.13104.

Brown, N., Buse, C., Lewis, A., Martin, D. and Nettleton, S. (2021a). 'Pathways, practices and architectures: Containing antimicrobial resistance in the cystic fibrosis clinic', *Health*, 25(2): 196–213. https://doi.org/10.1177/1363459319866894.

Brown, N., Nettleton, S., Buse, C., Lewis, A. and Martin, D. (2021b). 'The coughing body: Etiquettes, techniques, sonographies and spaces', *Biosocieties*, 16: 270–288. https://doi.org/10.1057/s41292-020-00196-3.

Bryder, L. (1984). 'Papworth Village Settlement–a unique experiment in the treatment and care of the tuberculous?', *Medical History*, 28(4): 372–390.

Bud, R. (2007). *Penicillin: triumph and tragedy*. Oxford: Oxford University Press.

Buse, C., Martin, D. and Nettleton, S. (2018). 'Conceptualising "materialities of care": Making visible mundane material culture in health and social care contexts', *Sociology of Health and Illness,* 40(2): 243–255. https://doi.org/10.1002/9781119499749.ch1.

Campbell, M. (2005). 'What tuberculosis did for modernism: the influence of a curative environment on modernist design and architecture', *Medical History*, 49(4): 463–488. https://doi.org/10.1017/S0025727300009169.

Calvillo, N. (2018). Political airs: From monitoring to attuned sensing air pollution. *Social Studies of Science,* 48(3), 372–388. https://doi.org/10.1177/0306312718784656

Chandler, C. (2019). 'Current accounts of antimicrobial resistance: stabilisation, individualisation and antibiotics as infrastructure', *Palgrave Communications*, 5, 1: 53. https://doi.org/10.1057/s41599-019-0263-4.

Colomina, B. (2019). *X-ray architecture*. Zurich: Lars Müller Publishers.

Connor, S. (2006) 'Building breathing space' in Bakke, M. (ed) *Going Aerial: Air, art, architecture*. Maastricht: Jan van Eyck Academie. 118–134.

Conway S. (2008) 'Segregation is good for patients with cystic fibrosis'. *Journal of the Royal Society of Medicine*. 101(1_suppl):31–35. doi:10.1258/jrsm.2008.s18007

Cooper, G. (2002). *Air-Conditioning America: Engineers and the controlled environment, 1900–1960*. Baltimore: Johns Hopkins University Press.

Dancer, S. (2013) 'Infection control in the post-antibiotic era', *Healthcare infection*, 18(2): 51–60. https://doi.org/10.1071/HI12042.

Douglas, M. (1966). *Purity and danger: An analysis of concepts of pollution and taboo*. Routledge & Kegan Paul.

Drake, S. (1997). 'The Architectural Antimephitic: Modernism and Deodorisation', *Architectural Theory Review*, 2(2): 17–28.

Escombe, A.R., Oeser, C.C., Gilman, R.H., Navincopa, M., Ticona, E., Pan, W., Martínez, C., Chacaltana, J., Rodríguez, R., Moore, D., Friedland, J. and Evans, C. (2007). 'Natural ventilation for the prevention of airborne contagion', *PLoS Medicine*, 4(2: 68.

Forty, A. (2003). 'The modern hospital in England and France: the social and medical uses of architecture' in King, A., (ed) *Buildings and Society.* London: Routledge. 39–57.

Fox, N.J. (1997). 'Space, sterility and surgery: circuits of hygiene in the operating theatre', *Social Science and Medicine*, 45, 5: 649–658. https://doi.org/10.1016/S0277-9536(96)00381-4

Garnett, E. (2020). 'Breathing spaces: modelling exposure in air pollution science', *Body and Society*, 26(2): 55–78. https://doi.org/10.1177/1357034X20902529

Gauvain, H. (1933). 'The Hastings popular lecture on sun, air, and sea bathing in health and disease', *The British Medical Journal*, 1: 57–61.

Gieryn, T. (2002) 'What Buildings Do'. *Theory and Society*, 31, 35–74. http://doi.org/10.1023/A:1014404201290

Hall, E.T. (1907). 'On Sanatoria'. *The Builders' Journal*, March 27, 138.
Hobday, R.A. and Dancer, S.J. (2013). 'Roles of sunlight and natural ventilation for controlling infection: historical and current perspectives', *Journal of Hospital Infection*, 84, 4:271–82. https://doi.org/10.1016/j.jhin.2013.04.011
Holmdahl, T., and Lanbeck, P. (2013). 'Design for the post-antibiotic era: Experiences from a new building for infectious diseases in Malmö, Sweden', *HERD: Health Environments Research and Design Journal*, 6(4): 27–52. https://doi.org/10.1177/193758671300600403
Irigaray, L. (1999). *The Forgetting of Air in Martin Heidegger*. Austin: University of Texas Press.
Jackson, M. and Fannin, M. (2011). 'Letting geography fall where it may – aerographies address the elemental', *Environment and Planning D: Society and Space*, 29: 435–444. https://doi.org/10.1068/d2903ed
Kembel, S. W., Meadow, J., O'Connor, T., Mhuireach, G., Northcutt, D., Kline, J., Moriyama, M., Brown, G., Bohannan, M., and Green, J. (2014) 'Architectural design drives the biogeography of indoor bacterial communities'. *PLoS ONE* 9(1): e87093. http://doi.org/10.1371/journal.pone.0087093.
Kisacky, J. (2017). *The Rise of the Modern Hospital: An architectural history of health and healing, 1870–1940*. Pittsburgh: University of Pittsburgh Press
Kisacky, J. (2005). 'Restructuring isolation: hospital architecture, medicine, and disease prevention', *Bulletin of the History of Medicine*, 79(1): 1–49. https://doi.org/10.1353/bhm.2005.0029.
Lande, B. (2007). 'Breathing like a soldier: Culture incarnate', *The Sociological Review*, 55(1_suppl): 95–108. https://doi.org/10.1111/j.1467-954X.2007.00695.x.
Latour, B. (2004). *Air*. www.bruno-latour.fr/sites/default/files/P-115-AIR-SENSORIUMpdf.pdf (accessed 18th Feb 2026).
Le Corbusier. ([1930] 1967). *The Radiant City: Elements of a doctrine of urbanism to be used as the basis of our machine-age civilization*. London: Faber and Faber.
Lefebvre, H. (1991). *The Production ofSspace*. Oxford: Blackwell.
Lorimer, J. (2020). *The Probiotic Planet: Using life to manage life*. Minneapolis: University of Minnesota Press.
Lowton, K. and Gabe, J. (2006). 'Cystic fibrosis adults' perception and management of the risk of infection with Burkholderia cepacia complex', *Health, Risk and Society*, 8, 4: 395–415. https://doi.org/10.1080/13698570601008263.
Macnaughton, J. (2020). 'Making breath visible: Reflections on relations between bodies, breath and world in the critical medical humanities', *Body and Society*, 26(2): 30–54. https://doi.org/10.1177/1357034X20902526.
Martin, D., Brown, N., Buse, C., Nettleton, S., and Lewis, A. (2025). 'An architecture of risk: How the past breathes in the design of future clinical space'. *Ephemera: Theory and Politics in Organization*. https://ephemerajournal.org/contribution/architecture-risk-how-past-breathes-design-future-clinical-space-0. Accessed 16th February 2026.
Mesman, J. (2009). 'The geography of patient safety: a topical analysis of sterility', *Social Science and Medicine*, 69, 12: 1705–1712. https://doi.org/10.1016/j.socscimed.2009.09.055.
Nieuwenhuis, M. (2016). 'Breathing materiality: Aerial violence at a time of atmospheric politics', *Critical Studies on Terrorism*, 9(3): 499–521. https://doi.org/10.1080/17539153.2016.1199420.

Noakes, C. J., Sleigh, P. A. and Khan, A. (2012). 'Appraising healthcare ventilation design from combined infection control and energy perspectives', *HVAC andR Research*, 18(4): 658–670. https://doi.org/10.1080/10789669.2011.592054.
Oxley, R. and Russell, A. (2020). 'Interdisciplinary perspectives on breath, body and world', *Body and Society*, 26(2): 3–29. https://doi.org/10.1177/1357034X20913103.
Papworth NHS Foundation Trust (2023). 'How we celebrated 75 years of the NHS'. 10 July 2023. https://www.royalpapworth.nhs.uk/our-hospital/latest-news/how-we-celebrated-75-years-nhs. Accessed 14th February 2026.
Prior, L. (1988). 'The architecture of the hospital: A study of spatial organization and medical knowledge', *British Journal of Sociology*, 39(1): 86–113. https://doi.org/10.2307/590995.
Prior, L. (1992). 'The local space of medical discourse', in Lachmund, J. and Stolberg, G. (eds.) *The Social Construction of Illness*. Stuttgart: Franz Steiner. 67–84.
Rousell, D., and Lupton, D. (2025). 'Atmospheric Wellbeing: Sensing the More-Than-Human Dynamics of Air', *Cultural Studies↔ Critical Methodologies,* 26(1): 3–13. https://doi.org/10.1177/15327086251387108.
Sloterdijk, P. (2004). *Spharen III*. Frankfurt: Suhrkamp.
Sloterdijk, P. (2009). *Terror from the Air*. Los Angeles: Semiotext.
Sommerville. T. (1960). 'The control of hospital infection'. *The Architects' Journal*, July 7, 132: 3403.
Swain, F. (2013). 'Fresh air and sunshine: the forgotten antibiotics', *New Scientist*, 220, 2947: 34–37. https://doi.org/10.1016/S0262-4079(13)62906-1.
Varrier-Jones, P. (1916). 'Tuberculosis and the working man, an appeal to friendly societies', *Cambridge Papworth Archives*, M 1–20: 9.
Varrier-Jones, P. C. (1930). 'The institutional treatment of tuberculosis'. *The Journal of State Medicine (1912-1937),* 38(5): 268–277.
Wagenfeld, M. (2008), 'The Aesthetics of Air: Experiments in Visualising the Invisible' Architectural Design, 78: 20–25. https://doi.org/10.1002/ad.669
Yaneva, A. (2022). *Architecture after COVID*. London: Bloomsbury Publishing.

PART III

Framing bodies and human health

Introducing

Elizabeth Shove, Cecily Maller and Simon Cohn

In some respects, the next two chapters belong in the previous section. They do so in that both deal with the place of 'the material' – including microscopic materials, infrastructures and the status of the human body. However, we group them together and discuss them separately because they revolve around a series of more specific questions about the social organisation of porosity (especially of the human body) and because both deal with matters of boundary-making and flow.

It is true they approach these problems from very different starting points. As will become clear, Blue (Chapter 8) provides a careful and useful review of somewhat abstract ideas about the place of the human body in practice theory. By contrast, Cohn (Chapter 9) presents detailed ethnographic accounts of the day-to-day 'work' of managing interpretations of care and contamination in contemporary hospital settings. Methodologically, the contributions are wide apart, but at the end of the day, they reach somewhat similar conclusions.

Reading between the lines, Cohn foregrounds the everyday ambiguity of concepts, categories and discourses. This is not incompatible with the parallel argument that distinctions are real in their effects and that at any one moment they orient the performances of different actors – nurses, parents, maintenance staff and more. The point of connection is that for Blue, the figures enacting interpretations like those Cohn describes (including definitions of care, dirt, risk etc.) represent momentary 'crossing points' through which materials and ideas flow and interact.

DOI: 10.4324/9781003685210-10

It is true that Cohn does not explicitly consider 'the body' or what more-than-human studies bring to practice theory, and it is also true that he puts forward a somewhat 'presentist' account: capturing a moment in what are evidently longer-term histories of germs, theories of infection and concepts of risk. This is consistent with Cohn's method of 'ethnographic' attention. To be clear, his approach does not necessarily exclude a more extensive narrative – as Cohn explains nurses routinely engage with a range of human and non-human 'materials'. However, different strategies are needed to produce accounts of practices and distinctions that stretch out over time. In other words, ethnographic attention, alone cannot generate the range of empirical material implied by the agenda that Blue sets out.

A related question has to do with the terms in which these two authors 'see' and describe processes of flux and flow over time. For Cohn, this is in essence a matter of representing moments in which specific distinctions are 'enacted' or made real in their effects, and of noticing how these vary and/or change. This is a pragmatic move. It is so in that making use of provisionally static categories enables (rather than undermines) an account of the ongoing reproduction of distinctions and their historical and spatial implications for definitions of people, microbes or other material arrangements. When read in this way, Cohn's studies provide some insight into the fine-grained detail of the processes and dynamics to which Blue alludes.

There are, of course, other possible interpretations. One is that Cohn's work exemplifies some of the limitations that Blue maps out. These include a tendency to represent distinctions and boundaries as these are 'performed' and enacted by human beings, acting in the present. For Blue, this is to focus on 'actors' and what they do, rather than on the practices and processes that pass through them. This brings us back to the methodological conundrum of how to 'see' change as it happens, how to show how practices and traces of them extend over time (for instance, epigenetically), and how to represent spatial extent and interaction. There are limits to what ethnographic studies can deliver (basically they miss the history), but this is not the only challenge.

On the ground people are recurrently involved in doing the boundary work associated with concepts of the body, health and risk, but for social theorists (and for Blue) the danger is that everyday categories reproduce dualistic traditions and versions of human exceptionalism. The puzzle of how to work with and also reject conventional concepts of the body is common to both. But again, both resolve this problem in different ways. Blue's response is more forthright. Because he focuses on practice theory (not on practices as they reproduced in different settings) he treats interpretations of the body as expressions and traces of past and present practices that prefigure some and not other futures. Discourses of human exceptionalism might be widespread, but the challenge is to take a step back from this and work through the implications of microbial flows for practice theory – never mind what happens in hospitals, homes or research laboratories. By contrast, Cohn, who is in the thick of the everyday worlds of care and infection control, draws on the multiple experiences of nurses, parents, estates staff etc. to reveal the contested and ambivalent character of boundary making on the ward, in the lobbies and in the public spaces of the hospitals he studied. In these worlds, there are strong versions of human exceptionalism (the body is treated as a real and bounded entity), but there are also more complicated accounts and everyday understandings of process and flow.

These are not the only points of overlap and tension. As readers will discover, both authors go along with the view that the margins of human and non-human bodies are porous, and both argue that this represents a point of connection between social, medical and biological sciences. For Cohn, or more accurately for those he studied, this is an ordinary feature of hospital life: in caring for new-born babies, nurses work with multiple technologies and objects, woven into ambivalent and dynamic narratives of care and control. As a matter of course they deal with 'leaky' bodies and with all manner of other movements, including those of air, of bacteria, of viruses and of water. As Blue explains, social theorists have been slow to catch up with these ideas, being wary of the dangers of biological determinism and the certainties of natural science. However, the problem, for Cohn and for Blue, goes beyond that of describing the impact of the biological on the social or vice versa. Instead, and for both, the more subtle task is to represent what Ingold refers to as biosocial configurations.

In taking this challenge to heart, both go along with the view that social practices are enacted by people, but never by people alone. From this, further questions follow, including questions about the passive and/or active status of the human practitioner (as performer, carrier or crossing point), and of the many non-humans involved, be they doors, tubes, viruses or water systems. Cohn's selection of cases and what he does and does not describe represents a way of organising relations of significance, and of positioning 'cases' in a certain light, often attuned to the project of representing the multiple positioning of 'the same' arrangements, and the overlapping of co-existing and not mutually exclusive way of seeing and doing. In this he draws attention to the (historical) organising of hospital life, and – implicitly – to how it is that 'beings of all kinds constitute each other's conditions of existence' (Ingold, 2011: 8). When read in this way, Cohn's chapter has the effect of filling out and illustrating some but not all aspects of Blue's position.

Blue's claim that bodies represent one of several processual media through which practices are reproduced and transformed is different, and distinctive, in that it focuses on the lives of practices, and the material arrangements (including human and non-human bodies) that they generate. By contrast, Cohn deals with the flip side of this equation – writing about how bodies (human and non-human) carry and enact distinctions and practices. In some ways this is an important theoretical difference, but in other ways it is no more, and also no less, than a matter of analytic approach.

In conclusion, Cohn's chapter is not simply an empirical 'application' of the sorts of ideas that Blue sets out. As this linking text makes clear, these two authors align and diverge in ways that go beyond differences of methodology and style. They share some ideas about social theory, microbes and the body, and on other counts they take a different course. The limits of both contributions reflect their different ambitions, but in putting them together we hope to ignite debates that travel in several directions at once. For some readers, a strong process orientation provides a means of bridging between past and present, and of understanding how multiple interpretations (boundaries and distinctions) co-exist and shape each other. For others, grasping the implications of these ideas depends on understanding what they mean on the ground, and in the everyday settings in which practices unfold and in which practitioners (human, non-human both) are constituted. This is not an 'either or' situation – as we have emphasised, there are significant divides but the pairing is justified in that arguments that underpin these two contributions have more in common than might at first appear.

Reference

Ingold, T. (2011). *Being Alive: Essays on movement knowledge and description.* London: Routledge. https://doi.org/10.4324/9781003196679.

8

PRACTICE THEORY AND THE BIOSOCIAL BODY

Stanley Blue

Introduction

The premise of this edited collection is that contemporary global health challenges – ranging from the geography and distribution of zoonotic diseases, the rise of antimicrobial resistance, and the accelerating consequences of climate change, to increasing rates of non-communicable conditions such as cardiovascular disease and type 2 diabetes – cannot be understood without attending to microscopic matter, including viruses, microbes, and cells. Such phenomena require socio-theoretical accounts that extend beyond the human and that encompass the biological, microbial and environmental. In short, the problems at stake are biosocial: made and remade through relations among bodies, infrastructures, ecologies and micro-organisms.

I take my cue from the proposition that practice theory offers a distinctive and productive method of conceptualising global health challenges by framing these as the outcome of intertwined biological, microbial and sociological processes. By taking practices as the principal organising heuristic, theories of practice provide analytic access to the discursive, material, spatial and temporal dimensions of social life – how they are constituted, organised, distributed and transformed. This orientation supports a shift away from dyadic accounts of human–environment or human–microbe relations towards an analysis of how everyday practices, which variously depend on plant, animal, human and technological life, develop trajectories and relations with other practices, generating wider effects that matter for the constitution of biosocial phenomena. Crucially, this provides a means of integrating microbes, bodies and environments into practice-theoretical explanation not as separate performers, carriers or contexts, but as integral

DOI: 10.4324/9781003685210-11

dimensions of social life that matter for the organisation and distribution of practical activity.

So far, practice theorists have had relatively little to say about microscopic or microbial dynamics, biologies or epigenetics. While there are notable exceptions (including Wakefield-Rann (2021), Maller (2018), Shove et al. (2026)) practice-theoretical work has been more fully developed in relation to fields such as organisational processes (for example the global organisation of risk management (Jarzabkowski et al., 2015)), technology and infrastructure (Shove et al., 2018) and environmental sustainability. In extending this work to contemporary global health challenges, practice theorists have much to learn from more-than-human approaches that foreground planetary, animal, microbial and environmental entanglements, and from biosocial accounts that recognise the inseparability of biological and social processes.

The central claim of this chapter is that integrating biological, environmental and microbial accounts with practice-theoretical ones requires a re-conceptualisation of the body of the practitioner. The chapter describes two analytical turns: first, from discrete, localised human and non-human 'encounters' to historically extended connections among shared social practices; and second, from a discrete and present practitioner to a horizontally and vertically extended, multi-dimensional practitioner conceived as the ongoing medium of becoming that underwrites the dynamics of practice.

Social theory and the body

The aim of this first section is not to offer a comprehensive history of how bodies have been understood in social theory, but to introduce a small number of influential positions that lie behind the terms in which practice theories conceptualise the body. Read together, these positions reveal recurring tensions around absence and presence, culture and biology, form and process and human and non-human life. These tensions help explain both the strengths and limitations of practice-theoretical approaches and point to the need for further conceptual development.

The absent body

A familiar claim in socio-theoretical accounts is that the body was largely absent from social theory until the late twentieth century. While this 'absent body' thesis (see Leder, 1990) captures an important shift of emphasis, it risks overstating the case. As Shilling (2020) and many others note, the body has never been wholly missing from social and philosophical thought: Marx's concern with labouring bodies, Durkheim's attention to ritual and Mauss's analysis of bodily techniques all testify to long-standing engagements with corporeality. Beyond sociology, phenomenological, philosophical and non-Western traditions have foregrounded the body in different ways.

What the absent body thesis captures is a disciplinary tendency within post-Enlightenment Western thought, namely, the relegation of the biological body to the natural and biomedical sciences. In sociology, this division was reinforced by efforts to distance social explanation from biological determinism, particularly in the aftermath of the Second World War and the exposure of eugenics programmes. As a result, biology came to be treated as analytically dangerous terrain, to be avoided rather than critically engaged with. This legacy entrenched a disciplinary division in which the body as organism was positioned outside the remit of social theory (see Pálsson, 2016).

The significance of this history is not simply that it represents a particular moment in which the body is neglected in social theorising, but that it demonstrates the endurance of this disciplinary inheritance. Even when the body later became a central object of analysis, assumptions about biology being external to the social continued to shape the terms in which embodiment was theorised.

The body as cultural object

By the 1980s and 1990s, the body had become a prominent object of sociological analysis, particularly within postmodern and cultural approaches. In this context, the body was understood primarily as a site of inscription: a surface upon which identities, hierarchies and distinctions were written, displayed and contested. Sociological attention focused on practices of bodily modification and presentation – such as fashion, dieting, cosmetic surgery and tattooing – as emblematic of broader cultural processes. However, this shift did not so much resolve the problem of the absent body as reconfigure it. While bodies were now highly visible, they were usually treated as symbolic objects rather than as living, material processes. As critics observed at the time (e.g. Davis, 1997), sociological accounts often appeared to privilege minds over bodies, imagining social power as operating through consciousness. The body was present, but largely as a passive substrate or bearer of meaning rather than as an active participant in reproducing the organisation of social life.

This orientation was reinforced by developments in the life sciences. The Human Genome Project, for example, reaffirmed the biological body as the domain of genetics and molecular biology. Even critical sociologists tended to focus on the cultural production of scientific knowledge, including genomics, rather than on developing alternative biosocial accounts. The result was a re-emphasis of disciplinary distinctions with social science attending to meaning and representation, leaving biology to claim the material body. For social theory, this sustained a conception of the body as discrete, individualised and 'skin-deep' – a view that practice theories seek to move beyond, but do not always escape.

The Living Body

Against interpretations of the absent body and of the body-as-object, pragmatist and phenomenologically informed approaches advanced a conception of the body as lived, skilled and active. Drawing on Merleau-Ponty and Mauss, these perspectives foregrounded the body as the site of practical knowledge and action: not a passive surface, but an active medium through which practices are enacted, learned and reproduced.

Bourdieu's concept of *habitus* (Bourdieu [1980] 1990) exemplifies this orientation. By locating durable social dispositions in embodied ways of moving, perceiving and acting, *habitus* positioned the body as central to social reproduction. The lived body became both the subject and object of action. This formulation is crucial for practice theories, many of which adopt embodiment as a foundational starting point rather than as a process requiring explanation.

At the same time, this emphasis has generated enduring questions. Critics, including Ingold (2023), have argued that theories of embodiment risk objectifying bodies and reintroducing dualism if embodiment is treated as a mechanism through which 'culture' is deposited in bodies. Strong practice-theoretical accounts following Bourdieu insist that learning is not a matter of internalisation but of participation: becoming skilled means moving from peripheral to fuller involvement in practices, as Lave and Wenger (1991) show.

While that position resolves some difficulties, debates about embodiment have continued to unfold against the backdrop of assumptions of biological fixity. The lived body might have been made active and social, but it was still implicitly bounded as present, individual and biological – an issue that has only recently come into sharper focus alongside developments in biological theory.

Plastic bodies

From the 1990s onwards, research in neuroplasticity, epigenetics and developmental systems has suggested that bodies are dynamic and responsive, shaped throughout the life course by social and material environments. This work has shown how diets, toxins, stress and socioeconomic conditions become biologically embedded, affecting gene expression and physiological development. As Meloni (2015) argues, these 'postgenomic' perspectives no longer treat genes and environments as separate factors that occasionally interact. Instead, environments are understood as active participants in biological development. Bodies are consequently thought to be permeable and impressionable from conception onwards, continually formed through their relations with social and material conditions.

Recognition of the plasticity of bodies has also challenged sociological accounts that have treated the body as absent or symbolic. These 'new biologies' have opened the possibility of genuinely biosocial analyses in which biological and social aspects are intertwined. For practice theory, these developments suggest that embodied dispositions are not merely socially learned but also biologically shaped over time. Equally, concepts of plasticity, alone, do not resolve questions about bodily boundaries or relations to environments.

More-than-human-bodies

More-than-human theories also challenge the centrality of the discrete human body in social analysis. Influenced by actor-network theory and new materialisms, these approaches decentre the human by recognising that bodies are assemblages composed of multiple other bodies, including microbes and cells, and entangled with infrastructures, technologies and environments. From this perspective, bodies are distributed and relational rather than self-contained. Scholars such as Maller (2018) argue that such approaches enable rethinking health and environments as outcomes of heterogeneous relations involving humans, animals, plants, microbes and technologies. Agency and vitality are treated as distributed across these relations rather than located solely in human actors. By foregrounding the multiple constituencies that make up any 'body', more-than-human approaches expand the analytic field, including entities previously imagined to be peripheral or inert.

However, important limits remain. While these approaches significantly correct human-centred analysis, they do not fully resolve how to conceptualise the subjects and objects of biosocial reproduction, nor do they explain how extended biological and social processes matter for each other over the longer run.

Biosocial bodies that are becoming

The move towards 'biosocial becomings', articulated by Ingold and Pálsson (2013), represents a decisive break with divisions between the biological and the social. Rejecting the assumption that forms precede processes, this perspective insists that beings are not pre-formed entities but trajectories of movement and growth. Bodies, in this view, are ongoing becomings, generated through biosocial relations that unfold over time rather than fixed objects upon which social or biological forces act.

Crucially, Ingold and Pálsson argue that the biological and the social are not complementary domains operating at different analytical levels but are inseparable and that there should be no division between them. Human becomings are entangled with the becomings of plants, animals, technologies and environments, all of which co-constitute the conditions of life. What this perspective adds to more-than-human approaches is a strong temporal and developmental emphasis. Bodies are not only extended horizontally across heterogeneous relations, but vertically across time, through processes of growth, inheritance and transformation.

The notion of biosocial becoming raises an important analytical challenge for social theories of the body and for practice theories as well. If bodies are ongoing, entangled and processual, how can relations of influence and transformation be specified – for example, in tracing disease transmission, environmental harm or uneven health outcomes? As the editors of this volume suggest, practice theory offers one possible way forward. However, I argue that any analysis that begins with practices must adopt a horizontally and temporally extended conception of both bodies and practices. The following section outlines the power, the potential and the limits of practice theory when dealing with biosocial phenomena.

The power, potential and limits of practice theoretical analyses

While other chapters in this volume introduce the core tenets of practice theory, and comprehensive accounts are readily available elsewhere (Schatzki, 2012; Nicolini, 2013; Shove et al., 2012), what matters for present purposes is the value of focusing on practices as a means of conceptualising processes of biosocial becoming. In taking up this challenge I do not simply rehearse what practice theory is but try to show that it offers a productive framework for analysing biosocial phenomena. In part, the answer lies in the potential to overcome a set of longstanding divisions in social theory, many of which were illustrated in the preceding discussion of how the body has been conceptualised.

By shifting attention away from individual persons and towards the extension and interconnection of practices across time and space (Giddens, 1984), practice theories reposition practices as the basic unit of social analyses. This move enables analysts to move beyond dyadic framings (e.g., agency and structure, mind and body, micro and macro) and instead examine how social activity is organised, distributed and transformed through ongoing configurations of practice.

Practice theory is not alone in seeking to unsettle binary forms of social analysis. Other approaches similarly challenge dualisms by emphasising expansive forms of action or subjectivity. What distinguishes practice theory, however, is its sustained use of the heuristic of practice as a nexus of doings and sayings (Schatzki, 1996). Practices are shared and embodied forms of practical activity and practical understanding, only partially ordered internally and dependent on their sequencing, synchronisation and interconnection with other practices. They are not bounded entities or cultural ideas that are 'embodied' by individuals, but open-ended configurations whose trajectories matter for how social, material and biological relations are organised over time.

This heuristic grants access to the material, discursive, spatial and temporal dimensions of the social as they matter for one another. Practices circulate, intersect, bifurcate and hybridise; they support each other's persistence or contribute to each other's decline (Shove, 2023). Infrastructures (that might be physical, biochemical, environmental or digital) are integral to these dynamics, sustaining and reshaping complexes of practice (Schatzki, 2002; Watson and Shove, 2022; Schatzki, 2019). Through their reproduction, practices also lay down economic, political, material and temporal architectures that connect them (Kemmis, 2019) and that shape future trajectories.

This conceptual vocabulary gives practice theorists powerful analytic purchase on contemporary health and environmental challenges. It allows phenomena such as antimicrobial resistance, uneven air quality or rising rates of obesity (Shove et al., 2026) to be analysed not as accumulations of individual choices or structural determinants, but as effects of interconnected practices unfolding across time and space.

Critically, however, constellations of practice exist only insofar as they are reproduced by people (Schatzki, 1996; Shove et al., 2012), which is why practice theorists insist on understanding action as embodied and practical. For this reason, realising the analytic potential of practice theory for global biosocial phenomena demands careful attention to the status of the body and embodiment.

As the next section shows, the way in which the practitioner is conceptualised, and the assumptions about embodiment that underpin different formulations, matter significantly for what practice theory can explain. My argument is that only by conceptualising the body of the practitioner as biosocial and extended can practice theory adequately address global health challenges shaped by biological, social and environmental entanglements.

Three figures of the practitioner (and of the body)

Within practice theories, the practitioner is the subject of action – the one who practices. This figure is not identical to the conception of the human body, but the two are inseparably connected: assumptions about the practitioner entail parallel assumptions about the body, and vice versa.

In showing what this entails I work through three figures of the practitioner exemplified in the works of Maller (2019), Reckwitz (2002), Schatzki (2017) and Shove (2012). These include the practitioner as *performer*, as *carrier*, and as *crossing point*.[1] Each figure highlights different aspects of the relation between practices and bodies, and each delineates distinctive analytical possibilities and constraints regarding issues of flux, flow and biosocial becoming.

The practitioner as performer

The conception of the practitioner as performer is perhaps the most familiar, but also perhaps, the most frequently misunderstood, figure in practice theory. The idea echoes Erving Goffman's dramaturgical account of social life (1959), in which human beings conduct themselves as if they were actors on a stage. Social roles, like theatrical scripts, provide patterns of action that are interpreted, enacted and performed in particular situations. In this dramaturgical sense, performance highlights both the structured nature of social life (dance, or drama) and the agency of individuals who carry out and adapt their roles, contributing to the life of the play.

Stronger uses of the concept of performance in practice theories draw more from the work of Judith Butler, and the idea of performativity (1990). For Butler, performances do not simply express pre-given roles; rather, they bring identities into being through repeated enactments. Practice theorists draw on this insight in arguing that while people perform shared practices, their performances are simultaneously shaped and constrained by the practices they enact. Schatzki captures this line of thought with the suggestion that performances 'befall' practitioners (Schatzki, 2010: 170): people do not stand outside practices and choose whether or how to perform them, but are themselves constituted through performance.

This performative framing has been used to question what looks like an anthropocentric bias in practice theories. For example, Maller and Strengers (2019) ask whether non-human beings (including pets, robots, fungi and viruses) can be said to 'perform' practices? In suggesting that non-humans participate in or co-constitute practices, these authors challenge the singular status of the human practitioner. Yet, in its simplest form, the performer figure also tends to anthropomorphise non-humans, treating them as interchangeable with humans on the stage of social life. Whether one speaks of a person, a pet or a robot performing a practice, the focus remains on the immediate act of enactment, framed as an interaction between a discrete subject and a practice.

Analytically, the figure of the practitioner as performer (whether human or non-human) privileges the moment of enactment, and the (variously constrained) agency of the performer. This positions variation in practices as a function of individual interpretation, choice or creativity. Broader historical and material dynamics (for instance, of pet ownership, breeding, and land use that might shape the dog walk) risk being side-lined as the context of contemporary performance. More sophisticated accounts of performativity, while attentive to repetition and history, frequently retain the assumption of a discrete subject and of his, her or its practices. In this respect, the performer figure restricts the analytic reach of practice theory, confining it to localised acts rather than including the constitution of social phenomena across time and space.

The practitioner as carrier

The second figure, the practitioner as carrier, exists alongside the figure of the practitioner as performer. Whereas the figure of the performer draws attention to the moment of individual enactment, the figure of the carrier shifts the focus to practices themselves (see Reckwitz, 2002). In this analysis people are conceived of as vehicles through which practices are sustained and reproduced. In this framing, agency does not lie with people but with practices, which are conceptualised as having their own trajectories and logics of development. While they are not passive or inert, practitioners, in this sense, are carriers who provide the energy and bodily presence that enable practices to endure.

This shift is crucial for realising the critical potential of practice theory. It makes it possible to grasp practices as dynamic social phenomena that compete, overlap and interact in organising the reproduction of social life. Practices require practitioners in order to survive, just as vampires require blood: they draw on the time, attention and bodily capacities of their carriers (Shove and Pantzar, 2007). From this perspective, people are indeed 'creatures of habit', but it is habits or more precisely, practices, that constitute the generative units of social life (Shove, 2012).

The figure of the carrier brings into view questions of recruitment, retention and defection. How are people drawn into new practices? What enables them to abandon old ones? What kinds of competences, material arrangements and embodied dispositions are necessary for recruitment to succeed? These questions are especially pertinent for analyses of health and environmental sustainability, where shifting participation in practices, including those that matter for diets, energy use or modes of transport, depends on and can have wide-ranging implications for all kinds of bodies and bodily resources, including the microscopic and microbial.

The carrier figure is intimately linked to the body in that carriers are corporeal beings whose embodied dispositions and physical capacities enable them to sustain some practices and not others. Embodied forms of competence, including driving, eating and working, anchor the reproduction of practices in bodily routines.

Analytically, the strength of the figure of the practitioner as carrier, lies in decentring individual subjectivity and providing a platform for focusing on the lives of embodied and shared practices. By inverting the relation between subject and object, however, the carrier figure risks reifying practices themselves, as if they were quasi-organisms with vitality somewhat independent of those who enact them. While this orientation is useful for analysing the reproduction and persistence of social life, it is less useful for explaining novelty and change. Because practitioners are viewed as carrier of practices, the, lively and extensive biosocial dynamics that emerge across human and non-human bodies and environments are cut out of the picture.

The practitioner as crossing point

A third figure is that of the practitioner as crossing point. This interpretation underlines the fact that practitioners never carry a single practice at a time but are always located at the intersection of multiple practices that traverse and constitute their lives. People are simultaneously practitioners of eating, commuting, parenting, working, exercising and countless other activities. The intersecting demands, rhythms, and temporalities of overlapping practices shape their lives (see Pred, [1990] 2019; Reckwitz, 2002).

This formulation broadens the analytic horizon. It draws attention to how practices bundle, compete and align in the organisation of everyday life. Recruitment into one practice may depend on participation in another; conversely, defection from one may free time, energy or resources for others. With the idea of crossing point, the adoption of cycling as a commuting practice is not a question of a relationship between the practice of cycling and a given person. Instead, the demography of cycling to work is conditioned by urban infrastructures, workplace cultures and household routines as well as competing demands for practices and schedules that might require flexibility, transporting cargo and other people.

Thinking of the practitioner as a crossing point consequently reframes the status of the human body involved in practice. In this case, the body is not an individual possession or a passive substrate, but part of a social body: a demographic, cohort or collective constituted by the intersection of multiple practices. Critically, the idea of the practitioner as crossing point positions the body of any one person as part of a social body, both the medium and outcome of intersecting practices – simultaneously shaped by, and shaping, the constellations of practices in which it participates. In effect, the idea of the practitioner as a crossing point, in attending to multiple practices, brings the subject performer and object carrier together.

The analytic significance of treating the practitioner as crossing point is to focus on how practices intersect and how their intersections distribute burdens and benefits across populations of practitioners. Rather than trying to study aspects of climate change by examining discrete performances of individual practices or by investigating how specific people or populations are recruited to specific practices, the conception of crossing point enables analysts to move from acquisition of embodied knowledge to the interaction and distribution of particular complexes of practices. In this way, the concept of a crossing point foregrounds the entanglement of practices across space and time. However, this formulation does not (empirically or as a matter of conceptual possibility) feature aspects of microbial, biological or ecological processes, nor does it show how crossing points change over time.

The three figures of the practitioner, as performer, carrier and crossing point, illuminate different ways in which practice theories conceptualise the relationship between practices, bodies and social life. Each provides distinctive analytic possibilities, but each also brings its own limitations.

In summary, the performer figure foregrounds enactment and reminds us that practices are realised only in performance. However, this emphasis risks narrowing analysis to discrete moments of action and interaction, privileging individual interpretation while neglecting broader material and historical dynamics. The body is largely absent.

The carrier figure decentres individual agency and emphasises the structuring and reproductive capacities of practices themselves. It provides powerful tools for analysing persistence, recruitment and defection, but tends to reify practices and leaves little scope for novelty and change. The body is the object and container, the vehicle for practices.

The crossing point figure offers the most expansive view of the three. By conceptualising individuals as simultaneously caught up in multiple intersecting practices, it extends the analytic horizon to the relations and conflicts between practices that shape social life. The body is social and shared, constituted at the intersection of practices and shared across cohorts. But it is present and, even though it is social, discrete in the sense that the crossing point remains the human practitioner.

These differences matter. How the practitioner is conceptualised shapes the questions practice theorists ask, the scope of the analyses they conduct and how they might frame challenges relating to health or the environment. By extending the figure of the practitioner through a less restrictive conception of the human body, practice theories and practice theoretical research enable more expansive accounts of the embodied, biosocial and more-than-human constitution of contemporary life.

Practice theory and the biosocial body

In bringing this chapter to a close I develop a revised conception of the practitioner as biosocial. Following Ingold and Pálsson's (2013) provocation that the social and the biological are not complementary domains but one and the same, the central task is to conceptualise the practitioner's body as more than a discrete, bounded organism. The notion of the biosocial is not without risks, particularly the danger of reducing the concept to a simple hybridity of biology and society. However, approached carefully, it offers a way of conceiving the practitioner as 'fully social': constituted through shared practices extended in time, entangled with non-human bodies and environments, and simultaneously the site and medium of biological and social processes.

The argument proceeds in three steps. First, drawing on recent developments in epigenetics and the developmental origins of health and disease, I show that practices are not only socially learned but materially embodied and inherited across generations. Warin et al.'s (2016) notion of (bio)*habitus* extends Bourdieu's concept of *habitus* by demonstrating how dispositions are sedimented not only in social histories but also in molecular and developmental ones.

Second, I move beyond questions of whether to 'add in' non-human bodies or simply decentre the human, and instead reconceptualise humans and non-humans as mutually constitutive developmental conditions. Ingold's (2011) adoption of 'developmental systems theory' (Oyama, 2000) for anthropology makes sense of how organisms, environments and technologies combine to form the matrices within which bodies grow, adapt and endure.

The final step returns to the figure of the practitioner, now reconceptualised as extended not only horizontally but temporally and trans-generationally. Understood as processual rather than performative, the practitioner corresponds to the shape of practice itself. Conceived in this way, 'the practitioner' opens new possibilities for analysing the historical and multi-dimensional relations through which biosocial phenomena are organised.

(Bio)Habitus

Bodily knowledge is typically understood as both the subject and object of action, the basis of practical competence and the medium through which it is enacted. The effect is that in practice theories, the practitioner is commonly conceptualised as a present set of embodied dispositions configured in, or mattering for, the subject. Framed in this way, analyses of practice tend to focus on a restricted set of questions: how practitioners perform, reproduce, negotiate or abandon practices; how they are recruited into or defect from them; or how practices shape and are shaped by particular bodies.

Even where practitioners are understood as multiple and as caught up in intersecting practices with long and entangled histories, the analytical focus is often fixed on the present because specific forms of embodied knowledge are imagined to live and die with the individual subject. While this does not amount to a simple disregard for the past, it limits attention to the timespan and remit of a single human life, treating longer histories as background conditions rather than as constitutive of the practitioner itself. One consequence is that practices appear as relatively stable constellations to which bodies are oriented in the present rather than as a medium shaped across generations.

Megan Warin and colleagues (2016) address this limitation through the concept of (bio)*habitus*. Drawing on developments in epigenetics and metabolomics (for more, see Meloni, 2019), alongside critiques of the nature-culture divide (Ingold and Pálsson, 2013), they propose a reformulation of habitus that fundamentally alters the status of the body. Rather than treating nature and culture, biology and society, as distinct explanatory domains, (bio)*habitus* conceptualises them as simultaneous and mutually constitutive. Bodies are thought to be shaped through layered biological and social histories that extend across generations.

In their work on rising rates of obesity, Warin et al. (2016) show how epigenetic inheritance complicates straightforward accounts of either biological or social lineage. From this perspective, the body is a biosocial medium stretched over time and shaped by lived, environmental and historical experience. In utero exposures, life-course conditions, and intergenerational effects all contribute to the embodied dispositions through which practices are reproduced and transformed at a collective level.

(Bio)*habitus* thus foregrounds what Warin and colleagues describe as an 'embedded body' (Warin et al., 2016: 15): one impregnated by its own past and by the social and material environments within which it develops, and therefore susceptible to change across evolutionary, developmental and transgenerational timescales. The analytic potential of this concept lies in its capacity to redirect attention from how practitioners enact practices in the present to how practices sediment into biosocial forms that endure across generations.

Because this particular work remains focused on human metabolism and obesity, there is a risk of re-inscribing the human body as the primary locus of practice-theoretical analysis. If we are to develop a biosocial practice theory, we need to go beyond the human, repositioning human and non-human bodies as mutually constitutive developmental conditions within which practices take shape.

Developmental conditions

More-than-human theories make it clear that 'the body', whether conceived as lived, embodied, shared, or stretched across time, is never exclusively human. Human biological bodies are composed of multiple other bodies, from cells and microbes to organ systems, and are extended through technologies, infrastructures and ecological relations. From this perspective, retaining a discrete human form as the primary site of social action skews analyses of phenomena that involve and include animals, viruses, plants, technologies and ecological systems.

This is not only a question of orientation but also of analytical scope. When the human body remains the primary locus of action, analysis tends to reproduce questions of influence and effect: how conditions shape human bodies, or how human bodies act back on conditions or other bodies. Even when the human body is understood as social and temporally stretched, as in Warin and colleagues' (2016) account of (bio)*habitus*, the underlying frame invites questions about how pre-existing conditions imprint themselves upon a given form. From this perspective, the body (even as biosocial media) remains something that is acted upon.

Ingold's (2023) critique of embodiment is central to this point. When human activity is analytically distinguished from the rest of life, there is a danger of reaffirming a model in which conditions act upon a form that then responds. Ingold's position (see for example Ingold, 2011) involves two related moves. First, he resists placing human action on a plane above or apart from other forms of life. Second, he rejects the suggestion that form precedes process. Together, these moves enable a re-conceptualisation of practices as matrices of developmental conditions that shape, and are shaped by, all forms of life they involve.

From this perspective, beings of all kinds constitute one another's conditions of existence across generations. Human activities establish conditions for non-humans, just as non-human organisms contribute to the growth and development of humans. Accordingly, practices can be understood heuristically as the configurations through which these developmental relations are organised and sustained.

This insight is crucial. It is so in that it suggests that bringing more-than-human conceptions of the body into view requires attention not to interconnected forms but to mutually constituting processes. The notion of developmental matrices makes it possible to reconceive practices as ongoing conditions of becoming – conditions that cut across humans, non-humans, technologies and environments alike. In this sense, practices are not performed upon bodies, nor merely carried by them, but are the very conditions through which bodies *of all kinds* are generated.

Ingold's account strengthens the case for extending (bio)*habitus* beyond the stretched human body and prepares the ground for a practice-theoretical analysis that decentres the human and foregrounds biosocial entanglements. The final step is to conceptualise the practitioner not as performer, carrier or crossing point, but as processual figure, stretched across time and space, biosocial in constitution and inseparable from these developmental matrices.

Processual practitioner

To articulate the image of a processual practitioner, one whose body is shared and social, extended over time and integrated with non-human bodies as part of mutually developmental conditions, it is useful to draw on developments in the philosophy of biology and connect these to arguments in practice theory about the 'extended practitioner' and the 'geometric shape' of practice.

In the philosophy of biology, John Dupré and colleagues have been at the forefront of a shift from conceiving of organisms as 'things' to understanding them as processes. Their argument is straightforward but radical: the basic building blocks of reality are not substances but processes. From this perspective, organisms, including human bodies, are not bounded objects but unfolding processes that only appear stable when captured in a momentary 'time slice'.

This turn to process resonates strongly with Ingold's critique of form and with Warin et al.'s concept of (bio)*habitus*. Each insists that bodies, human, animal or microbial, should not be treated as discrete entities but as entangled and ongoing processes. Consider a virus, typically imagined as a fully assembled and infectious particle existing outside a host cell. From a processual view, the viral life cycle depends on, and contributes to, the mutual conditions that sustain it, including its hosts. For process philosophers, the persistence of any organism or form depends on the stability of these conditions. As Dupré and Nicholson argue, it is the spatio-temporal organisation of processes and their relations to other processes that ground persistence and causal power.

Nicholson and Dupré explain:

> The spatio-temporal organization of a process and its spatio-temporal and causal relations to other processes determine its persistence and stability, and are also what grounds its properties and causal powers.
>
> *(Nicholson and Dupré, 2018: 13)*

In other words, practices persist, not because of the actions of discrete practitioners, but because they are sustained through the entanglement of spatio-temporal relations and conditions. The body of the practitioner, in turn, is a processual medium through which practices are reproduced and transformed.

A similar orientation to the figure of the practitioner appears in Wallenborn's (2013) account of 'Extended Bodies and the Geometry of Practices', in which the subject of practice theory is described as the 'passage of successive extended bodies' (Wallenborn, 2013: 199). Drawing on feminist technoscience and theories of material extension, Wallenborn argues that human evolution and social life are inseparable from the development of technologies and infrastructures. From this position, he develops an account of extended bodies that are 'hybridised' in particular ways, and that carve out overlapping topographies that together constitute the geometric shape of practices.

If Wallenborn's account of extended bodies is brought together with Warin's (bio)*habitus* and Ingold's emphasis on developmental conditions, it is obvious that 'the practitioner' is not bounded by skin or confined to the timespan of an individual life. It is a processual concept: a biosocial body stretched across time, constituted through developmental matrices and extended through material and technological assemblages. Its persistence depends on the organisation and distribution of practices, which are themselves stabilised through biosocial, environmental, microbial and technological processes.

Seen in this way, the reproduction of all bodies, human and non-human, living and non-living, can be imagined as processes stabilised by the social organisation of practices.

Conclusion: A biosocial practice theory needs a conception of the biosocial body

This chapter has argued that bringing practice theories to bear on contemporary global health and environmental challenges, depends on first developing an account of the figure of the practitioner and the body in practice theory. Global problems such as climate change, antimicrobial resistance, zoonotic disease and the rise of non-communicable conditions cannot be adequately understood through approaches that keep the biological and the social separate, nor through analyses that confine themselves to discrete performances or to presentist accounts of embodied knowledge. To appreciate the enduring, cultural, technological, microbial and ecological processes at play requires a conception of the body that is processual, and extended across time and space, technologically and biologically.

This conception of the biosocial body has several implications for practice theory in general and for those that make use of the figures of the practitioner as performer, carrier or crossing point, or some combination of the three. First, it emphasises the need to focus on longer timescales. A processual conception of the practitioner makes clear the necessity to not be beholden to the lifespan of individual practitioners and to include intergenerational and evolutionary processes in explanations of biosocial phenomena. Second, it decentres the human without reducing non-humans to anthropomorphic performers, instead positioning all bodies, human, animal, microbial, technological and environmental, as mutually constitutive processes. Third, it repositions the practitioner not as the subject of practice but as the processual medium and outcome of practices, the temporary stabilisation of extended bodies through which practices persist and change.

For global health and environmental research, these moves matter. They make it possible to show how practices (of food production, health care, forms of daily living, etc.) contribute to the spread of antimicrobial resistance, not simply by tracing behaviours of individuals, but by following the developmental matrices of microbial, technological and social processes. They make it possible to understand the intergenerational dynamics of obesity not as competing questions of lifestyle choice or genetic inheritance, but as the indeterminate, embodied effects of (bio)*habitus* formed across histories of diet, metabolism, and textures of social life (Martínez et al., 2020). And they make it possible to attend to issues of environment and climate change not only in relation to the consumption choices of individuals or the policies of states, but as processes that are always entangled with other mutually conditioning human and non-human processes.

The conclusion, then, is that a biosocial practice theory requires a biosocial body. By integrating insights from epigenetics, developmental systems theory, more-than-human approaches and process philosophy, practice theory can leave behind the defined figure of the practitioner and the distinct, separate biological body to develop a richer account of the entangled, processual, and extended constitution of social life.

Note

1 These 'figures' do not represent the detail of any one account, but rather stand in for representations of how the conceptualisations of the practitioner and the body are taken up in practice theories and research that develops those ideas.

References

Bourdieu, P. ([1980] 1990). *The Logic of Practice.* Translated by Richard Nice. Cambridge: Cambridge University Press. https://doi.org/10.1017/CBO9780511812507.

Butler, J. (1990). *Gender Trouble: Feminism and the subversion of identity.* London: Routledge. https://doi.org/10.4324/9780203824979.

Davis, K. (1997). *Embodied Practices: Feminist perspectives on the body.* London: Sage.

Giddens, A. (1984). *The Constitution of Society: Outline of the theory of structuration.* Cambridge: Polity Press.

Goffman, E. (1959). *The Presentation of Self in Everyday Life.* New York: Knopf Doubleday Publishing Group.

Ingold, T. (2011.) 'Prologue: Anthropology Comes to Life' in Ingold, T., *Being Alive: Essays on movement knowledge and description.* London: Routledge. https://doi.org/10.4324/9781003196679.

Ingold, T. (2023). 'A Breath of Fresh Air: Or, Why the Body Is Not Embodied', *SubStance*, 52(1): 100–107. https://doi.org/10.1353/sub.2023.a900536.

Ingold, T. and Palsson, G. (2013). *Biosocial Becomings: Integrating social and biological anthropology.* Cambridge: Cambridge University Press. https://doi.org/10.1017/CBO9781139198394.

Jarzabkowski, P., Bednarek, R. and Spee, P. (2015). *Making a Market for Acts of God: The practice of risk-trading in the global reinsurance industry.* Oxford: Oxford University Press.

Kemmis, S. (2019). *A Practice Sensibility: An invitation to the theory of practice architectures*. London: Springer. https://doi.org/10.1007/978-981-32-9539-1.
Leder, D. (1990). *The absent body*. Chicago: University of Chicago Press.
Lave, J. and Wenger, E. (1991). *Situated Learning: Legitimate peripheral participation*. Cambridge: Cambridge University Press. https://doi.org/10.1017/CBO9780511815355.
Maller, C. (2018). *Healthy Urban Environments: More-than-Human Theories*. London: Routledge. https://doi.org/10.4324/9781315620534.
Maller, C. (2019). 'Dynamic Bodies in Theories of Social Practice: Vibrant Materials and More-than-Human Assemblages' in Strengers, Y. and Maller, C. (eds.) *Social Practices and Dynamic Non-Humans: Nature, materials and technologies*. London: Springer. 87–107. https://doi.org/10.1007/978-3-319-92189-1_5.
Maller, C. and Strengers, Y. (2019). *Social Practices and Dynamic Non-Humans: Nature, materials and technologies*. London: Springer. https://doi.org/10.1007/978-3-319-92189-1.
Martínez, A., Anduro, I. and Bojorquez, I. (2020). 'The Biohabitus of Scarcity: Bio-Social Dispositions and the "Obesity Epidemic" in Mexico', *Sociology of Health and Illness*, 42(5): 1095–1107. https://doi.org/10.1111/1467-9566.13080.
Meloni, M. (2015). 'Epigenetics for the Social Sciences: Justice, Embodiment, and Inheritance in the Postgenomic Age', *New Genetics and Society*, 34(2): 125–151. https://doi.org/10.1080/14636778.2015.1034850.
Meloni, M. (2019). *Impressionable Biologies: From the archaeology of plasticity to the sociology of Epigenetics*. London: Routledge. https://doi.org/10.4324/9781315169583.
Nicholson, D., and Dupré, J. (2018). *Everything Flows: Towards a processual philosophy of biology*. Oxford: Oxford University Press. https://doi.org/10.1093/oso/9780198779636.001.0001.
Nicolini, D. (2013). *Practice Theory, Work, and Organization: An introduction*. Oxford: Oxford University Press.
Oyama, S. (2000). *The Ontogeny of Information: Developmental systems and evolution*. Durham, North Carolina: Duke University Press. https://doi.org/10.1215/9780822380665.
Pálsson, G. (2016). 'Unstable Bodies: Biosocial Perspectives on Human Variation', *The Sociological Review Monographs,* 64(1): 100–116. https://doi.org/10.1002/2059-7932.12015.
Pred, A. ([1990] 2019). *Making Histories and Constructing Human Geographies: The local transformation of practice, power relations, and consciousness*. London: Routledge. https://doi.org/10.4324/9780429044649.
Reckwitz, A. (2002). 'Toward a Theory of Social Practices: A Development in Culturalist Theorizing', *European Journal of Social Theory,* 5(2): 243–263. https://doi.org/10.1177/13684310222225432.
Schatzki, T. (1996). *Social Practices: A Wittgensteinian approach to human activity and the social*. Cambridge: Cambridge University Press. https://doi.org/10.1017/CBO9780511527470.
Schatzki, T. (2002). *The Site of the Social: A philosophical account of the constitution of social life and change*. Philadelphia: Pennsylvania University Press.
Schatzki, T. (2010). *The Timespace of Human Activity: On performance, society, and history as Indeterminate Teleological Events*. Lanham, Maryland: Lexington Books. https://doi.org/10.5040/9781978737358.

Schatzki, T. (2012). 'A Primer on Practices', in Higgs, J., Barnett, R., Billett, S., Hutchings, M., and Trede, F. (eds.) *Practice-Based Education: Perspectives and Strategies*. Leiden: Sense Publishers. 13–26. https://doi.org/10.1007/978-94-6209-128-3_2.

Schatzki, T. (2017). 'Practices and People', *Teoria e Prática Em Administração*, 7(1): 26–53. https://doi.org/10.21714/2238-104X2017v7i1-32735.

Schatzki, T. (2019). *Social Change in a Material World: How activity and material processes dynamize practices*. London: Routledge. https://doi.org/10.4324/9780429032127.

Shilling, C. (2020). 'Embodiment', in Kivisto, P. (ed) *The Cambridge Handbook of Social Theory: Volume 2: Contemporary Theories and Issues*. Cambridge: Cambridge University Press. 249–271. https://doi.org/10.1017/9781316677452.014.

Shove, E. (2012). 'Habits and Their Creatures', *The Habits of Consumption: COLLeGIUM: Studies across Disciplines in the Humanities and Social Sciences,* Vol. 12: 100-112. Helsinki Collegium of Advanced Studies. Available at: http://hdl.handle.net/10138/34225.

Shove, E. (2023). *Connecting Practices: Large topics in society and social theory*. London: Routledge. https://doi.org/10.4324/9781003275107.

Shove, E., Blue, S. and Kelly, M. (2026). *Practice Theory and the Biosocial: Microbes, matter and milieu*. Oxford: Berghahn Books. https://doi.org/10.3167/9781836953395.

Shove, E. and Pantzar, M. (2007). 'Recruitment and Reproduction: The Careers and Carriers of Digital Photography and Floorball', *Human Affairs*, 17(2):154–67. https://doi.org/10.2478/v10023-007-0014-9.

Shove, E., Pantzar, M. and Watson, M. (2012). *The Dynamics of Social Practice: Everyday life and how it changes*. London: Sage. https://doi.org/10.4135/9781446250655.

Shove, E., and Trentmann, F. (eds.) (2018). *Infrastructures in Practice: The dynamics of demand in networked societies*. London: Routledge. https://doi.org/10.4324/9781351106177.

Wakefield-Rann, R. (2021). *Life Indoors: How our homes are shaping our bodies and our planet*. London: Springer. https://doi.org/10.1007/978-981-16-5176-2.

Wallenborn, G. (2013). 'Extended Bodies and the Geometry of Practices', in Shove, E. and Spurling, N. (eds.) *Sustainable Practices: Social theory and climate change*. London: Routledge. 146–164. Part of: https://doi.org/10.4324/9780203071052.

Warin, M., Moore, V., Davies, M. and Ulijaszek, S. (2016). 'Epigenetics and Obesity: The Reproduction of *Habitus* through Intracellular and Social Environments', *Body and Society,* 22(4): 53–78. https://doi.org/10.1177/1357034X15590485.

Watson, M. and Shove, E. (2022). 'How Infrastructures and Practices Shape Each Other: Aggregation, Integration and the Introduction of Gas Central Heating', *Sociological Research Online*, 28(2): 373–388. https://doi.org/10.1177/13607804211055495.

9

MICROBES AT LARGE IN THE HOSPITAL

Challenging concepts of care, contact and contamination

Simon Cohn

Introduction

This chapter focuses on the threat of microbes in medical settings, and on some of the attempts made to control them. Microbes have long been framed as enemies of human life and health – agents of disease that need to be eradicated, or at least curtailed. Modern medicine and public health have both been built upon this antagonistic relationship, from Pasteur's germ theory (Bordenave, 2003) to contemporary protocols of sterilisation and infection control (Kubde et al., 2023). Despite their sheer diversity, the potential to become entangled with human bodies and disrupt them has often propagated a generalised conceptualisation of infection, and a common range of strategies to combat them. Central to this are three straightforward assumptions; that the human body has some kind of integrity; that hazardous microbes normally exist elsewhere but pose a risk to health when they are proximal; and consequently, that the boundary between the body and a microbe, or the medium in which its carried, is a site of vulnerability where a breach might take place. A common approach is therefore simply to keep microbes at bay, or, if that is not possible, to ensure that boundaries are sufficiently robust and impermeable to prevent a potential 'chain of contamination' (Dancer, 1999).

The result is a highly spatialised depiction of microbial infection, utilising ideas of vectors, routes, pathways and colonisation to isolate different places from one another and depict how microbes thereby move between them. This not only demarcates the human body from its environment, but also what is considered biologically relevant from what is simply considered background or context (see for example, Diez Roux and Aiello, 2005). But

DOI: 10.4324/9781003685210-12

while this mechanistic approach has proven highly productive and effective across many areas of medicine, extending it uncritically to all domains of biomedical practice is not without consequence. One clear example is in the field of public health, where diseases at the population level are often modelled through this lens by treating variables as discrete, stable entities. Such representations necessarily have to bracket off relational accounts of social life that emphasise contingency, emergence and the ways health outcomes are enacted through specific socio-material arrangements, in order to pursue causal links between discrete entities.

However, applying this mechanistic approach to microbes and human–microbial encounters is also increasingly at odds with a number of contemporary scientific perspectives (Wakefield-Rann, 2021). Disciplines such as microbiology and immunology now tend to portray the relationship between humans and microbes as much more dynamic and context-dependent (Silverstein, 1991). In the majority of instances, the incursion of pathogens does not automatically lead to ill health, but is influenced by such things as microbial load or toxins produced as metabolic by-products (Parija, 2023), as well as the age, vulnerability and broader circumstances of the infected person (Russell, 2013). Indeed, many pathogens only cause significant disease when immunity is already compromised, for example, by a pre-existing health condition or attempts to treat it. Attending to these individual and contextual factors thereby challenges any simple, generalisable account of microbial infection, and the idea that transmission and contamination are a straightforward, linear matter. Nominating microbes as the primary discrete cause of many diseases may well be useful in some instances, but the danger is that other elements and practices rapidly fall by the wayside, while the microbes themselves become divided off from the local world they inhabit, the interactions that shape them, and the environments they create.

This way of thinking has also been taken up by recent scholarship in the social sciences which emphasise how microbes are not simply external threats, but active participants in the constitution of social life (Paxson, 2008; Lorimer, 2017). Both actor-network theory (Latour, 2005; Callon, 1986) and practice theory (Shove et al., 2012; Shove, 2017) invite us to see social order as emerging from heterogeneous relations, rather than as the exclusive domain of human actors. More-than-human approaches insist that entities such as microbes, materials, and infrastructures possess their own kind of agencies which inevitably become entangled with human ones (Haraway, 1989). Consequently, sites such as hospitals, households, farms, and urban environments are not simply backdrops against which microbial life unfolds but are actually constituted through ongoing negotiations with microbial presence and absence (Hinchliffe, 2017). And equally, specific practices such as handwashing, cooking or prescribing antibiotics are not merely technical interventions, but social acts that both respond to existing entanglements of humans and microbes as well as inescapably foster new ones.

Through such framings, microbes are not presented as simply biological adversaries, but highly significant actors whose presence destabilises neat boundaries between such things as nature and culture, the individual and collective, and indeed the microbe and the host (Brives, et al., 2021). Rather than existing outside of social life, they co-produce the very spaces, activities and infrastructures by which things like health and illness are defined, while their potential to be harmful, or indeed helpful, can never be solely attributed to specific characteristics and capacities they may have, but also from the multitude of arrangements they enter in to with other things (Wakefield-Rann et al., 2020). The never-ending flow of new encounters and interactions therefore challenges the more classic hygienic practices which strive to identify and intervene on divisions between where microbes are, and where they should not be.

This chapter describes how, despite the emergence of these more dynamic and dialogical understandings of human–microbial relations, a mechanistic framing of infection and infection control continues to operate within the field of hygiene and sanitation, precipitated by quite categorical ideas of health and disease (see for example, Schellack et al., 2016). It considers how the overriding concern with routes of transmission, surfaces and boundaries are sustained through a range of routines and practices. Two related concerns derived from this linear worldview shape medical activity: first, that infection control should focus on continuously identifying all possible routes of microbial transmission; and second, that controlling an infection ultimately depends on preventing any breaches of boundary along those routes. By illustrating how this is done, the chapter shows how understandings of microbial risk emerge from the ongoing and repeated activities by diverse actors, and how this shapes what are considered possible or appropriate forms of response.

Hospitals offer a good site to explore these issues because, for the duration a patient is the subject of direct medical care and intervention, they are also the site of intensified microbial awareness. Practices of hygiene in a hospital frequently reproduce the spatial logic through work to either demarcate, separate or contain. Although every individual action and event may well all appear unique if one focuses on the care of a particular patient, the reality of hospital life is that it is a place dominated by repetition and routine. Different professional roles not only have their set of everyday jobs and duties to perform, but also oversee different kinds of spaces: some staff act directly on the interior of the patient; others interact with a patient while they are lying in a bed or sitting in a chair; while other hospital workers are involved in activities to maintain the fabric of the building or the complex infrastructure required for it to function. All of these tasks bring people, things and microbes into particular configurations, and with this, a concern for particular boundaries – whether directed to the surface of the skin, the air that is breathed in or the water that is ingested. Considerable effort is consequently focused on maintaining borders and introducing barriers to avoid possible infection across these overlapping sites; material objects, consumables, hospital protocols and procedures are continuously employed to avoid unnecessary contact and control the flow of things that may carry pathogens.

The solution to control infections in a hospital, however, can never be as simple as the elimination of contact. Medicine is also infused with the idea that good doctoring and good nursing requires proximity and touch (Davin et al., 2019). Contact not only conveys empathy and intimacy but the dissolving of an unkind divide between the carer and the cared for, which is often seen to have a central therapeutic value in itself (Rosa et al., 1998). Even on occasions when physical touch is not possible for some reason, apparently innocuous and trivial utterances can nevertheless convey a partial sense of this mutuality and closeness (Cocksedge et al., 2013). So, whilst hygienic practices may be concerned with eliminating or controlling direct contact between things through the maintenance of boundaries, other medical practices promote convergence and the blurring of barriers as an essential aspect of care. Medicine is thereby inherently paradoxical: constantly creating divisions and categories, yet also seeking to connect and traverse such distinctions. Both are ways of doing health work, whether the primary concern is with contamination or a concern with care, and both position boundaries as key sites of attention and the place where a great deal of medical activity gets done.

Having conducted research in National Health Service (NHS) hospitals over a number of years, I have observed this tension on many occasions – whether directly alongside patients, during regular multidisciplinary meetings held by various specialist teams across the organisation, or simply following the daily routines of individual staff members. Across all of these encounters, practices of hygiene and methods of mitigating infection were routine aspects of medical activity, often conducted with very little reflection or deliberation. They are built into the roles of different staff members, the arrangements of wards and other hospital areas, the design of clinical equipment, the provision of consumables, and the various ways in which all the different kinds of waste are disposed of. Below, I draw on these accumulated observations to illustrate how different types of professional jurisdictions and their accompanying knowledges determine what people do and the things with which they interact. By describing examples in which boundaries and spaces become the focus of activity, the chapter shows how human–microbial entanglements in healthcare are produced through multiple, overlapping practices, whose coexistence frequently generates tensions and competing priorities.

Skin as boundary

One of the most controlled areas in the hospital where patients are considered especially vulnerable are the neonatal wards. Here, the environment must be meticulously controlled for light, sound, and temperature. A baby's exact location in the area, established after an early clinical assessment, can signal further levels of vigilance that may be necessary. Compared to looking after new-borns with minor complications in the larger postnatal recovery areas, staff looking after those on the dedicated high-intensity ward have to follow far stricter protocols to address increased vulnerability. One perimeter follows another, ensuring that there are multiple barriers preventing any microbial ingress. Staff and visitors must adhere to strict instructions before entering, including handwashing, the wearing of masks and gowns, the removal of jewellery, how many people are allowed in at one time and what physical contact is permitted. Movement in and out of the ward is tightly regulated, with doorways and access points leading onto coloured floor markings that demarcate safe and unsafe zones, and who exactly is permitted to cross them. Even a gloved hand or a shared pen carries potential microbial contamination. At the centre, of course, is a fragile and susceptible body. Lying in a transparent incubator, a baby is frequently administered prophylactic antibiotics under the assumption that all contact carries potential danger.

These physical demarcations are replicated in the allocation of distinct professional jurisdictions, with specific individuals having their own dedicated tasks. There is always at least one neonatal consultant, together with other neonatologists, paediatricians or specialist doctors providing round-the-clock support. Most of the routine work, however, is done by specialist nurses, who are assigned just one or two of the new-born babies to ensure constant oversight. Surfaces are continually wiped before and after every contact: even the rhythm of touch is shaped by vigilance. When a nurse opens the hatch of an incubator to reposition the baby or adjust a line, he moves deliberately and with practiced economy because less movement equates to fewer chances for microbial invasion. Nothing is casual, and everything is repeated time and time again. Incubators, ventilators and other medical technologies must be maintained in sterile conditions while thermometers, catheters and syringes are either single-use or have to be put into dedicated containers to be sent to the Hospital Sterilisation and Disinfection Unit. Even objects such as bed sheets and blankets are implicated in the same microbial concern.

Yet the drive to maintain aseptic conditions represents only one aspect of the work conducted. The delivery of fluids, nutrients and medication are just as essential, continually challenging any goal of complete hygienic enclosure. Rhythms of feeding, washing, and monitoring therefore repeatedly disrupt the static spatial arrangements. As a result, other practices are organised around cautious access, rather than total separation, each carried out according to highly prescribed and carefully choreographed patterns that establish how boundaries may be momentarily opened, managed and then re-sealed.

In such settings, when so many technologies are physically connected to the new-born, the boundaries of the body are often not self-evident. Attachments such as feeding tubes, oxygen sensors and ventilator piping blur any obvious sense of bodily limits. Whilst this ambiguity may initially be a visual one, the equipment itself is often the focus of medical activity and attention just as much as the new-born inside an incubator. Multiple practices thereby extend across the assemblage, creating extended boundaries of care and microbial concern. In this way, the body as co-constituted by human and non-human actors is not a theoretical but an evidently practical reality, derived from the work of the specialist nurses and others working in the unit. In fact, it extends even further into spaces beyond the unit, enlisting other staff, such as the specialised technicians and engineers responsible for the repair and maintenance of the sensitive equipment. Acknowledging this distribution through the roles of numerous staff not only disrupts conventional notions of patienthood, but also which boundaries and surfaces are the most significant for potential microbial contamination: paradoxically, the logic of protection through containment is extended into numerous spaces via the different tasks conducted to keep the baby alive.

Once a new-born is well enough to be moved from this high-intensity care unit to the more general neonatal ward, the significance of policing boundaries shifts. In apparent contrast to the many protocols directed at ensuring all forms of contact are kept completely sterile, practices such as touching, positive handling and the promotion of breastfeeding might initially appear contradictory. For example, it is not uncommon to see a mother encouraged by staff to sit in a chair, gown loosened, with a tiny infant pressed against her bare skin. Here, rather than trying to avoid all contact per se, the work of nurses and others shifts to enabling particular *kinds* of contact to take place. This has increasingly become a significant aspect of clinical practice, with the aim of collapsing certain boundaries, not shoring them up. Instead of focusing on whether a particular surface is sterile, or having to execute an isolated procedure, staff increasingly attend to how various things come into contact with one another. But rather than opposing the concern with pathogens, they are instead a development of it: alongside such things as bodily warmth and sensing the breathing or heartbeat of another, their purpose is to facilitate microbial exchange. The new-born baby – now sufficiently robust to have been transferred into this area of the ward – is also deemed to be well enough to begin to have a range of microbial encounters, and through them, become more vigorous and independent.

The point is that when clinical routines and practices are directed to simply keeping a vulnerable new-born alive, microbial infection is a totalising concern, foregrounding actions to police protected spaces and secure impenetrable territories as much as possible. But, if the baby survives beyond this period and can be detached from the machines that were directly essential for its survival, medical practices shift to encouraging certain kinds of interactions and promote greater extensions into the world. Part of this process is to become entangled with microbes and the cultivation of various bodily systems in order that the baby can continue to grow and thrive. And whilst one may interpret this as an account of child development, it is possible to find similar parallels in other specialist areas and units of the hospital. For example, intensive care units are highly concerned with maintaining a sterile environment while patients are critically vulnerable; but if a patient improves and is moved out to a high dependency unit or directly to a general ward, not only are these concerns relaxed, but they are replaced by a new emphasis on practices that encourage the body to regain independence by means of contact and interaction with other people and things. By attending to connections, flows, and linkages, the porosity of bodily boundaries starts to emerge as significant, precisely as the patient becomes healthier – because, ultimately, the management of that porosity is itself a quality of health.

The body, as an object of medical attention, is not a given but is constituted through those boundaries that come to be considered most significant. As these boundaries extend outward, encompassing microbial risk across other surfaces and spaces, the body is enacted at multiple scales and through the involvement of diverse actors.

Beyond the body

Although an obvious task of hospital work is to shield patients because many are especially vulnerable, many are actually carriers of harmful microbes themselves, threatening the health of others. Moreover, hospitals provide conditions that can readily support microbial proliferation: they accommodate patients with compromised immunity, maintain warm environments, contain damp and concealed spaces, and involve numerous potential human and material carriers. As a result, hospital spaces are continually being made and remade, shifting to manage areas of risk or danger. During an outbreak of norovirus in one hospital, for example, the main revolving entry doors were resolutely locked with a sign stuck on the glass warning outsiders of the emergency. Visitors and non-essential staff all walked up to the entrance and were forced to turn back. But there were similar signs across various pinch-points inside the building as well, preventing people from moving from one designated area to another. The goal was clearly one of containment, but although the signage implied that people were the potential carriers of the virus around the hospital, the real effect was to halt the interactions that might occur, and the multiple ways in which microbes might be able to actively take part in them.

While the work of doctors and nurses is largely directed to looking after their individual patients, a specialised team focuses on these broader risks across the hospital, and the movement of microbes at a collective, institutional level. Their work is to identify specific events and places where there may be a particular risk. This Infection Control Team oversees ongoing monitoring of potential outbreaks, manages how the hospital should deal with patients who may be carriers, and implements a range of hygiene policies and cleaning regimens.

The first infection control initiatives were introduced in the middle of the last century in response to outbreaks of staphylococcal infections, particularly in surgical and maternity wards. Previously, the responsibility for hospital hygiene largely fell to ward matrons, the nurses under their management, and hospital orderlies (Forder, 2007). At this time, hygiene practices were largely taken to be a professional rendering of domestic ideas of cleanliness and tidiness, focusing on visible distinctions between clean and dirty, sterile and contaminated, inside and outside. Recognising the need for more systematic surveillance techniques to prevent outbreaks led to the creation of specialist infection control nurses, and eventually the rise of modern multidisciplinary teams which now include infectious disease consultants, microbiologists, and representatives of the hospital such as from the Estates department or Procurement. Importantly, this development is one that has paralleled evolving scientific and epidemiological techniques which make microbial risks visible in new and different ways. The rise of antimicrobial resistance (AMR), hospital acquired infections, and most recently the impact of COVID-19, has decisively established Infection Control as a pivotal specialism of the contemporary hospital.

The modern Infection Control team makes regular rounds and get to know other staff, the building and its infrastructure in very particular ways. Although the core members are trained nurses, their medical gaze now includes things like the taps, the air-conditioning vents and the coving edges where hospital flooring curves up the walls as places where possible threats may lurk. In doing so, the team generate a different set of significant boundaries to other hospital staff through the range of practices that they perform. And the truth is, despite depictions of hospital that suggest a carefully orchestrated approach to microbial risk, with increasing levels of cleanliness and restriction as one moves from the public to more clinical zones, the reality of many British hospitals undermines this. Most are a patchwork of architectural epochs, the result of decades of expansion, retrofitting, and reconfiguration. Corridors and passageways introduced for more efficient movement may lead to cramped, outdated rooms, while modern fixtures, such as new basins and toilet facilities, are frequently connected up to antiquated plumbing systems. The result is an agglomeration of areas and regions, edges and joins, across which things move around in unpredictable ways, forever complicating the goal of controlling the flow and accumulation of microbes.

Perhaps the most conspicuous signal of spatial concern are the hand sanitisers, accompanied by large and insistent warning notices, that mark entrance-ways throughout the building. Every staff member, patient, and visitor is instructed to stop at the door and use an antimicrobial gel – this has now become such a familiar expectation that there is real concern many people don't bother any more. The issue is not merely that an apparently inconsequential lapse may lead to a vulnerable patient gaining a serious infection, but that the very practice itself usefully marks out spaces of difference as people, and the things they bring with them, stop to comply, before then proceeding. On one occasion, the lack of working hand sanitisers at the entrance to some of the general wards led to quite a turmoil. For the ward staff, their use represented a tangible guarantee that all the other hygiene protocols were being upheld as well, and that the risk of pathogens was being taken seriously. So, their absence triggered unease, not merely because the boundary of the ward had been compromised, but also the sense of order and neatness as to what should be done where.

It is all too apparent that efforts to control microbes by either keeping things apart or controlling exactly how and when things should be in contact across the hospital is never straightforward. Fleshy, leaky bodies can never be fully contained. This is an obvious concern when it comes to the loss of blood or other body fluids from a physical injury, or when a syringe must be inserted into tissue, or locating a catheter into a patient's cavity. Infection Control may demand that the localised space has to have a 'deep clean'. This involves cleaning staff manually wiping and sterilising all surfaces with chemical disinfectants to ensure no pathogens remain. In addition, if there was a case of a particularly worrying infection, the use of ultra-violet light may be advocated, in which case the space has to be emptied and sealed, with warning signs placed outside while a tall lamp unit on a trolley is positioned inside and left on for half an hour or more. The high-intensity UV light not only reaches all the exposed surfaces but also any microscopic matter in the air itself. Rather than remove dirt, or fluids, or microbial matter, it works by shattering the DNA and RNA of microorganisms so they cannot reproduce or infect.

But clearly these strategies cannot be applied across the whole hospital, even though the droplets that people exhale, the sweat they exude, the faeces and urine they excrete, all move and circulate. Hospitals, just like individual patient bodies, are porous. Things need to move in and out all the time; patients, visitors, clinical staff, ancillary workers, managers, medications, equipment, food, drink. This continual flow means that the hospital composition is always changing, as communities of people, things and microbes, move throughout the fabric of the building. The many hygiene routines by which staff attempt to manage microbes may shape how hospital spaces are delineated and ordered, yet these arrangements are always partial, because hospitals are not stable entities but open assemblages of people, technologies, materials and infrastructures.

Because the dynamic interactions between these elements cannot be fully controlled, the possibility of microbial incursion is never eliminated. Infection Control therefore responds to a continual flow of assessments and adjustments that mirror the flow of threats: staff respond to patient histories, laboratory results, environmental swabs and reports of unusual cases as and when they arise. Rather than aiming for definitive containment, management at the scale of the hospital is organised through prioritisation – deciding which risks, spaces, and pathways demand the most attention at any given moment. Hygiene, in this sense, is an adaptive practice, defined as much by what cannot be governed as by what can. This produces a persistent tension between efforts to stabilise space by specifying what should happen where, and the constant movement of people, objects, air and fluids which are essential to hospital life. Boundaries may well be temporarily strengthened around a piece of equipment, a patient's bed, or an entire ward, but doing so long-term can obstruct other care practice. In this way, the tension between containment and contact that structures microbial concern at the bedside is replicated through different practices at the scale of the hospital itself.

Not everything can be bounded

The circulation of air within a hospital presents a particular challenge to any attempt at microbial containment. Whilst there is always a threat of pathogens from the outside coming in, there is just as much effort made to ensure air-borne microbes don't simply circulate inside. Draft seals on doors, air curtains, and the use of positive pressure rooms in critical areas, all exemplify efforts to try and govern microbial movement. In more modern hospitals, windows cannot open, and the flow of air is controlled using a system of ducts and vents to ensure heat isn't continuously lost. But air, by its very nature, resists straightforward confinement, especially when the movement of people and things is essential for the hospital to function. The very possibility of microbial presence in the air determines a wide range of actions and decisions, introducing new priorities that potentially clash with those held by staff who don't see such risks.

Take one instance in which the door to a particular ward never quite clicked shut easily. Instead, it had to be pulled behind you with just the right amount of force – firm, but not too sharp – or it would gently swing back open, stopping a few centimetres ajar. Everyone working on the ward soon acquired the knack, but most visitors were frustrated when it didn't latch and either pulled too hard or didn't bother at all. Although multiple maintenance requests had been logged to fix it, and someone had once come and made a few adjustments, the problem persisted. The issue was that the door was slightly sagging on its hinges with age, the frame somewhat warped by years of heavy use. For clinical staff already balancing large caseloads, the door was just another example of the infrastructure not quite working, but not really broken enough to matter. But for Infection Control, the issue wasn't simply an ageing door; the unsealed entrance was a potential route for airborne pathogens to spread. At a joint meeting, someone from Estates, in an exasperated tone, outlined the cost of a complete replacement, the backlog of repairs, and the impossibility of redoing every door in the building. It simply could not be a priority. In response, an Infection Control nurse reiterated the principles of isolation, containment, the issue of air movement, and how important it was to ensure everything was done to avoid an outbreak. The difference in priorities was not simply due to the distinct roles each had, but that the maintenance team simply saw the problem as a mundane repair of the door and its frame, while for Infection Control it was not the wood, but the incessant gap of air around it that was the focus of concern. Eventually, it was agreed that a temporary sign should be fixed to the door, asking everyone to 'Please ensure door closes fully'. The paper quickly became grubby, curling at the corners.

Management of water within hospitals raises similar challenges to boundary maintenance. NHS policies mandate rigorous controls for water safety, from temperature regulation to prevent the growth of Legionella, to routine microbial testing. In high-risk areas, sterile water is not only used for drinking, but also for washing and bathing immunocompromised patients. But the amassing of plumbing fixes and augmentations over the years complicates attempts to know where or how to intervene if a problem should arise; old lead piping, outdated cistern tanks and hidden water routes co-exist with modern plumbing and sterilisation equipment. 'Dead-legs' in the pipework (sections that see little or no water flow) may harbour stagnant water, while any maintenance activity might actually disturb sediments and introduce new contaminants. If waterborne microbial threats do emerge, such as traces of Legionella identified somewhere in the network, investigations must painstakingly work backwards – not only spatially, but often historically – to retrace the source and pathway of contamination within a system that may only be partially mapped.

One particular incident highlighted the difficulty of ensuring new systems could be safely integrated with old. A series of modern, sensor-activated water fountains were installed across one hospital so that people – especially patients sitting in waiting areas – would be able to help themselves. Within days, however, staff noticed small puddles on the floors beneath the spouts.

Ostensibly, the problem was that the jets released water unpredictably, so if cups weren't held at just the right angle or distance, water would spray out and land on the floors. For Estates, who had overseen their installation, this was just a teething problem with the mains-fed water pressure, which varied throughout the hospital as different pipe networks had been connected in an ad hoc fashion over the years. For Infection Control, however, the problem was not just the splashes, but what the puddles might then foster. Wet surfaces and residual moisture are potential microbial reservoirs where pathogens can quickly reproduce and be carried around across the hospital. For a while, the new water dispensers were shut off until a fix was agreed. A sense of exasperation accompanied the realisation that almost all improvements that might be made in the hospital would probably always create new opportunities for microbes to flourish.

Recently, some NHS hospitals have gone so far as to remove sinks entirely from specific areas, replacing water-based practices with antiseptic wipes, gels, and dedicated bowls that can be emptied and sterilised (Inkster et al., 2024). The shift reflects growing recognition that basin traps and drains can act as reservoirs for harmful microbes, and that splashes and water aerosols can disperse pathogens onto nearby surfaces, equipment, and into adjacent clinical areas. Biofilms that develop within pipes are particularly resilient: even with routine cleaning and disinfection, microbes can rapidly recolonise, rendering conventional hygiene measures insufficient (Hopman et al., 2017). This shift to 'water-free care' illustrates how concerns about circulation, contact and contamination are continually renegotiated. What was once assumed to be fundamental to hygiene practices is now being questioned, not because hand washing itself is seen as ineffective, but because once microbial life is traced a bit further beyond a delineated activity, the spill-over of one specific practice can be shown to create risks elsewhere.

Air and water pose particular challenges for containment not simply because they flow and fluctuate, but because they are indispensable to both patient survival and the everyday functioning of the hospital. They cannot be excluded or eliminated; instead, they must be continuously incorporated into practices of care and control. As a result, efforts to manage boundaries and organise space are persistently challenged by the very flows that hospital activities require. Through everyday practices, material objects, infrastructures and people are enrolled to regulate circulation in specific ways – for example through sealed doorways, zoning protocols, or plumbing systems – but this work is never complete because there is never a stable whole that can be fully enclosed or circumscribed. The broader point that has been made is that hospitals are sites of continual movement and circulation, while boundaries are always local sites in the making – that never fully encompass one space from another.

Conclusion

This chapter began by outlining how dominant ideas of hygiene draw on spatial conceptualisations and linear models of transmission, from which boundaries are identified as critical sites of microbial risk. Given that preventing and controlling infection underpins much of the activity within a large hospital, it might therefore be assumed that these ideas can be straightforwardly mapped onto hospital spaces. However, a focus on practice makes clear that hospital life is organised less by abstract categories or theoretical knowledge, and more by the routinised activities of many different members of staff. Because much of medicine is directed towards the individual patient, the body is treated as a key site of microbial vulnerability and the object of intense attention. This generates complex and varied actions, often enrolling an expanding range of staff, materials and practices, which effectively extend the body's boundaries outwards. In so doing, attention also spreads to microbial encounters across numerous contexts, and sometimes the entire hospital.

Of course, microbes have always been collaborators in the organisation of modern medicine, ranging from the design and layout of hospital wards, the implementation of handwashing protocols, and the formation of distinct professional jurisdictions. Yet hospitals are not simply clinical spaces; they bring together a wide range of people, roles and material objects whose purposes do not always align neatly with the formal goals of medicine. Hospitals are also places where people eat lunch, wait, pass time, socialise, work, wash, repair, transport goods and carry out countless routine tasks that sustain the building. The result is that what gets taken to be significant borders or edges of things is never fixed but always enacted through practices, meaning distinctions between such categories as clean and dirty, safe and risky, patient and environment, or indeed clinical and nonclinical, always emerge from specific doings and sayings. On occasions, different staff activities may well reinforce the same divisions, producing institutional coherence and relatively stable boundaries. But at other times, they intersect or even contradict one another, producing frictions and difference. Trying to control infections through a focus on spaces and boundaries consequently requires continual negotiations, both in terms of deliberations between varied hospital staff, and the wide range of material objects that emerge as significant.

At the beginning, I also introduced the idea that, at a conceptual level, there must be an inevitable tension between hospital practices of microbial control and those of care, which promote closeness and contact. This represents a particular manifestation of a broader contrast between frameworks that treat microbes as external threats to bounded human bodies, and bioscientific and social theories which increasingly describe human–microbial relations as dynamic, mutual and context-dependent. At first glance, the strategies seem to stand in opposition – one seeking to contain or exclude, while the other promotes interaction and intermingling. But as the examples from everyday hospital life show, competing interpretations rarely surface in direct conflict with each other like this. Microbial management and patient care are deeply entwined concerns, meaning that practices such as washing, changing linen or swabbing skin are simultaneously about microbial control *and* the expression of intimacy and respect. Although both are always present, the relative priority given to each depends on what forms of knowledge and objects of concern are foregrounded on any particular occasion.

Thus, although we might see the work of the Infection Control team as a form of localised biopolitics by governing bodies and hospital populations through particular knowledges of microbial risk (see Brown et al. Chapter 7), its effectiveness depends not only on discipline and exclusion, but also on relational practices between bodies, surfaces, infrastructures, and the microbes themselves. By paying close attention to the small, often overlooked details of how staff navigate their specific duties within the broader system, everyday moments reveal the complexity and interdependence of hospital practices, far beyond any formal job description. They show that infection control is not the application of fixed principles to stable environments, but an ongoing, situated accomplishment in which microbial risks and appropriate actions are continually made and remade, and in which any designated space or boundary is always provisional. The flow of microbes thereby endlessly complicates the tidy oppositions on which infection control protocols rest. Far from being passive, microbes act by disrupting and reconfiguring arrangements: they traverse surfaces, bodies and infrastructures, undermining spatial and categorical separations and pushing clinical practice to attend to flux, relation and movement. Thus, while strategies of containment and elimination may still be deemed necessary, they are always provisional and incomplete.

Just as infection is not a single, bounded event but an emergent outcome of multiple, distributed actions, so too are activities that may alter its occurrence. Recognising this opens up a more sustainable mode of microbial governance: one that accepts contingency, embraces improvisation and foregrounds practices of living *with* microbes, rather than against them. Ultimately, the hospital is not a battleground between medicine and microbes, but a site of ongoing negotiation between multiple forms of life and value. Care, in this setting, is about managing those interactions and heterogeneous associations, rather than trying to contain or eliminate certain things in order to protect others. As part of this, Infection Control work is revealed to be not merely the application of technical procedures, but a profoundly social and more-than-human activity, through which microbial and human agencies are mutually constituted.

References

Bordenave, G. (2003). 'Louis Pasteur (1822–1895)', *Microbes and infection*, 5(6): 553–560. https://doi.org/10.1016/S1286-4579(03)00075-3.

Brives, C., Rest, M. and Sariola, S. (2021). 'Introduction: From witnessing to withnessing' in Brives, C., Rest, M. and Sariola, S. (eds.) *With Microbes*. Mattering Press. www.doi.org/10.28938/9781912729180.

Callon, M. (1986). 'The sociology of an actor-network: The case of the electric vehicle' in Callon, M., Law, J., and Rip A. (eds.). *Mapping the Dynamics of Science and Technology: Sociology of science in the real world* London: Palgrave Macmillan. 19–34. https://doi.org/10.1007/978-1-349-07408-2_2.

Cocksedge, S., George, B., Renwick, S. and Chew-Graham, C.A. (2013). 'Touch in primary care consultations: qualitative investigation of doctors' and patients' perceptions', *The British Journal of General Practice*, 63(609): p.e283. www.doi.org/10.3399/bjgp13X665251.

Dancer, S. (1999). 'Mopping up hospital infection', *Journal of Hospital Infection*, 43(2): 85–100. www.doi.org/10.1053/jhin.1999.0616.

Davin, L., Thistlethwaite, J., Bartle, E. and Russell, K. (2019). 'Touch in health professional practice: a review', *The Clinical Teacher*, 16(6): 559–564. https://doi.org/10.1111/tct.13089.

Diez Roux, A.V. and Aiello, A.E. (2005). 'Multilevel analysis of infectious diseases', *Journal of Infectious Diseases*, 191(Supplement 1): S25–S33. https://doi.org/10.1086/425288.

Forder, A.A. (2007). 'A brief history of infection control-past and present.', *South African Medical Journal*, 97(11): 1161–1164.

Haraway, D.J. (1989). 'The biopolitics of postmodern bodies: constitutions of self in immune system discourse', *differences 1*(1): 3–43.

Hinchliffe, S. (2017). 'More than one world, more than one health: Re-configuring inter-species health' in Herrick, C. and Reubi, D. (eds.) *Global Health and Geographical Imaginaries*. London: Routledge. 159–175.

Hopman, J., Tostmann, A., Wertheim, H., Bos, M., Kolwijck, E., Akkermans, R., Sturm, P., Voss, A., Pickkers, P. and vd Hoeven, H. (2017). 'Reduced rate of intensive care unit acquired gram-negative bacilli after removal of sinks and introduction of "water-free" patient care', *Antimicrobial Resistance and Infection Control*, 6(1): 59.

Inkster, T., Walker, J. and Weinbren, M. (2024). 'Water-free patient care: a narrative review of the literature and discussion of the pressing need for a way forward', *Journal of Hospital Infection*, 152: 36–41. https://doi.org/10.1016/j.jhin.2024.06.006.

Kubde, D., Badge, A.K., Ugemuge, S., Shahu, S. and Badge, A. (2023). 'Importance of hospital infection control', *Cureus*, 15(12). https://doi.org/10.7759/cureus.50931.

Latour, B. (2005). *Reassembling the Social: An introduction to actor-network-theory*. Oxford: Oxford University Press. https://doi.org/10.1093/oso/9780199256044.001.0001.

Lorimer, J. (2017). 'Parasites, ghosts and mutualists: A relational geography of microbes for global health', *Transactions of the Institute of British Geographers*, 42(4): 544–558. https://doi.org/0.1111/tran.12189.

Parija, S.C. (2023). *Textbook of Microbiology and Immunology*. Berlin: Springer.

Paxson, H. (2008). 'Post-pasteurian cultures: The microbiopolitics of raw-milk cheese in the United States', *Cultural Anthropology*, 23(1): 15–47. https://doi.org/10.1111/j.1548-1360.2008.00002.x.

Rosa, L., Rosa, E., Sarner, L. and Barrett, S. (1998). 'A close look at therapeutic touch', *JAMA*, 279(13): 1005–1010. https://doi.org/10.1001/jama.279.13.1005.

Russell, P.S. (2013). *Clinical Approach to Infection in the Compromised Host.* London: Springer. https://doi.org/10.1007/978-1-4615-2490-8.

Schellack, N., Ismail, H. and Babarinde, O. (2016). 'Revisiting the principles of infection control', *SA Pharmaceutical Journal*, 83(6): 33–38.

Shove, E. (2017). 'Matters of practice' in Hui, A., Schatzki, T. and Shove, E. (eds.) *The Nexus of Practices: Connections, constellations, practitioners*. London: Routledge. 167–180. https://doi.org/10.4324/9781315560816.

Shove, E., Pantzar, M. and Watson, M. (2012). *The Dynamics of Social Practice: Everyday life and how it changes*. London: Sage. https://doi.org/10.4135/9781446250655.

Silverstein, A.M. (1991). 'The dynamics of conceptual change in twentieth century immunology', *Cellular Immunology*, 132(2): 515–531. https://doi.org/10.1016/0008-8749(91)90047-f.

Wakefield-Rann, R. (2021). *Life Indoors*. Singapore: Springer. https://doi.org/10.1007/978-981-16-5176-2.

Wakefield-Rann, R., Fam, D. and Stewart, S. (2020). 'Microbes, chemicals and the health of homes: Integrating theories to account for more-than-human entanglements', *BioSocieties*, 15(2): 182–206. https://doi.org/10.1057/s41292-019-00147-7.

PART IV

Ideas and implications for research and policy

Elizabeth Shove, Cecily Maller and Simon Cohn

The chapters in this section foreground fundamental questions about how paradigms and forms of knowledge configure the unequal interplay of microbes, people and policy interventions. Although they approach the task in very different ways, both authors show how groups and organisations mobilise ideas about infectious agents and diseases, and both show how interpretations of the microbial and the medical sustain some, but not other types of intervention.

Having said that, the style of analysis, and the scope of enquiry is really very different: Meloni (Chapter 10) deals with the long reach of Galenic notions of balance, noticing parallels between concepts of humours and more recent accounts of microbiomes. By contrast, Kelly and Shove (Chapter 11) work with a specific case, focusing on the UK government and its response to COVID-19 in 2020 and a year or two beyond.

To elaborate, Meloni identifies some of the risks attached to currently fashionable, post-microbial theories of balance, arguing that epigenetic legacies persist and that social groups that have suffered 'insults' in the past are, or might be forever excluded from contemporary interpretations of well-being. In effect he argues that epigenetic characteristics accumulate over time, and that the potential to live up to a template of 'good' gut health, or to have a well-ordered microbiome – is socially skewed. This begs further questions about how such a template arises, and whose interests it serves.

Kelly and Shove are more straightforwardly critical of the sorts of models of infection, and especially the focus on the 'R' value (or rate of reproduction), that dominated UK government policy responses to COVID-19. In this case, the claim is that conventional epidemiological models are founded on a handful of assumptions that systematically obscure social

DOI: 10.4324/9781003685210-13

gradients and differences, and that overlook decades of social research. As described, government advice to isolate, home school or maintain social distance exacerbated existing inequalities as did the tendency to consider 'the virus' apart from coexisting health conditions, and aside from the specific conditions in which it had deadly effect.

As both chapters show, theories of balance, or of viruses and how they spread, are integral to the reproduction of social difference. This is important in that ideas about disease, and about bodies and health, are performative – meaning that they are real in their effects, and that they matter for interventions and how these are framed.

In the case of COVID-19, dominant methods reproduced a medical model in which diseases are thought to have specific causes (the virus), and in which sources of infection are considered one at a time, and apart from the worlds in which they have effect. In theory, concepts of balance are more holistic, generating more complex accounts of dysfunction and threat. But in both cases, traditions and ways of thinking about infection and health overlook the inscribed consequences of past harms, disregarding the differential effects of long-term changes, including in diet, agriculture, ventilation, air quality and more.

Implicitly, both chapters suggest that there are alternative ways forward, and that it might be possible to escape these traps. For example, Meloni suggests that there could be scope for forms of biopolitical repatriation, that is for interventions that help level the playing field and enable 'balance' for all. Of course, this is to accept and work with a notion of 'balance' that is itself normative, but for Meloni, the point is that there is scope for debating and re-defining the meaning of this category. For Kelly and Shove, the challenge is to create forms of governance and politics that can handle and exploit different forms of theory and 'evidence', including that produced by the social sciences.

Whether these are plausible futures or not, the common conclusion is that debates, policies and forms of intervention are always and inevitably loaded. For practice theorists, the further conclusion is that dominant discourses – whether of balance, or of transmission – are part of and not separate from the histories and lives of policy making, the effects of which feed into, and in part constitute, the phenomena on which they focus.

10

DYSBIOTIC TIMES

Life in distress and the politics of knowledge in microbiome research

Maurizio Meloni

Introduction

The terms *dysbiosis* and, to a lesser extent, *eubiosis* (or even *normobiosis*) have become increasingly used in medical microbiome research over the last fifteen years (Hooks and O'Malley, 2017). They are used as umbrella terms to describe what can be defined as failed (the Greek root *dys*) versus good (*eu* in Greek) or *well-balanced* microbiome functioning.

For example, in the Planetary Health literature, dysbiosis, or life in distress, is framed as a 'global health issue' (…) 'a critical target in overcoming the health challenges of the twenty-first century' (Logan et al., 2016: 1). The notion of a 'dysbiotic drift' is also introduced to supplement the hygiene hypothesis – the *absence* of traditional early-life microbial exposure being viewed as cause for the rise of allergies, asthma, or autoimmune diseases. In this context, the term 'dysbiotic refers to the long-term trend toward unhealthy or chronically ill life connected with the ubiquity of westernised lifestyle and exposures "such as environmental contaminants, unhealthy diets, food additives, advanced glycation end-products and circadian disruptions" ' (Logan et al., 2016: 16).

Typically, a healthy or eubiotic microbiota is defined by its high diversity and lack of environmental or lifestyle disruption. Whether in humans or plants, it is, to use another term in the literature 'correctly assembled' (Paasch et al., 2023). On the other side, a dysbiotic microbiota is characterised by loss of beneficial microbes, reduction in diversity and overgrowth of pathobionts (Logan et al., 2016).

DOI: 10.4324/9781003685210-14

Triggers of these changes are often seen as environmental or lifestyle disruptions such as exposure to xenobiotics, poor hygiene or unhealthy diet. Consequences include metabolic, inflammatory and auto-immune diseases. For the human gut microbiota, diet is indicated as one 'such factor which can be used as a key regulatory component' (Nag et al., 2023: 68).

In a series of insightful articles, philosopher of biology Maureen O'Malley and colleagues have been highlighting the most visible shortcomings in the definition and operationalisation of these concepts in microbiome medical research. Hooks and O'Malley have, for example, argued that vagueness, circularity and confusion between causation and correlation in the usage of eubiosis and dysbiosis 'may affect how microbiota research develops from an association-focused science into a more fine-grained explanatory science' (Hooks and O'Malley, 2017: 1; Brüssow, 2020).

In their analysis of over 9,000 PubMed abstracts using the term 'microbiota', Hooks and O'Malley note, in particular, the preponderant usage of the term 'imbalance' to convey the notion of dysbiosis: for instance, in one of the articles they analysed, dysbiosis is defined as 'an imbalance in the microbiota composition and a shift in their function from normal to disease' (Kim et al., 2013: 6). Balance, more generally, is used in 3% of all ca. 160.000 articles in microbiome research (O'Malley, 2024). In a later essay, Sumrall and O'Malley (2024) moved the criticism to another level, suggesting uncanny resemblances between premodern humoral medicine (with its notions of balance and imbalance) and dysbiosis/eubiosis in current microbiome research.

It is not the first time that findings in postgenomic[1] disciplines have been compared to wider premodern or even non-Western (for lack of better terms) medical cosmologies, including humoralism, based on the leading power of environmental factors, the permeability of the human body and an emphasis on lifestyle as conducive to health (see for epigenetics: Meloni, 2019). In Sumrall and O'Malley however, the effect is double edged. These authors applaud the renewed connection of health and environment that a return to Galenism would bring, but also denounce a certain 'conceptual malaise in microbiome research' for its uncritical reliance on outdated scientific concepts (Sumrall and O'Malley, 2024: 11). In this chapter I wish to contribute to this debate on notions of balance and imbalance in contemporary microbiome research with an emphasis on *biopolitical* relevance rather than on epistemological confusion. I have a genealogical goal: if at least in certain sections of the medical literature, contemporary health crises are framed in terms of dysbiosis and its solution (eubiosis), it is important to have a detailed sense of the history of these concepts: there might be meanings or cultural templates that are buried in these notions that might need to be brought out into the open. This is significant because the issue of injured or distressed life sits at the intersection of two dramatically growing trajectories: increasing evidence of catastrophic stressors (both ecological and social) particularly on vulnerable populations, and realisation of the unique porosity of biological matters and their potential to become impressed, with lasting effects, by historical events and social structures, including racial and colonial violence.

The family tree of eubiosis and dysbiosis (a larger album)

While highlighting the central contribution, post WWII, of German microbiologist and nutritional scientist Helmut Haenel in the first systematic use of the terms dysbiosis and eubiosis, Hooks and O'Malley briefly outline an earlier history pointing to a triad of authors before WWII: Russian/Ukraine pioneer of immunology Élie Metchnikoff (d. 1916); US inventor, novelist and physician Elliot Furney, who used both terms in his utopian technoscientific novel *Culture, A Modern Method* (Furney, 1891); and finally, one generation later, German veterinary physiologist Carl Arthur Scheunert (d. 1957), who used the term *Dysbiose der Darmflora* in 1920 in relation to alterations in the intestine flora of horses (Scheunert, 1920; Hooks and O'Malley, 2017). As Hooks and O'Malley claim:

> We suggest that although these three authors provide very different resources for thinking about dysbiosis, their contributions nevertheless ended up being combined historically: Metchnikoff urged scientists to think about normal and abnormal microorganismal effects on hosts, Furney promoted the words dysbiosis and eubiosis but gave them a rather dubious fictional context, and Scheunert brought together the terminology and relevant microbe-host research.
>
> *(Hooks and O'Malley, 2017: 2)*

As with any genealogy, it is often our presentist need to find a clear family history that links these three authors, otherwise so different in goals, context, and scope of research. Moreover, Metchnikoff never used either eu- or dysbiosis, while calling attention to normal and pathological microbial effects on human health. Furney is the only one who uses both terms in his *Culture, a Modern Method* where he defines eubiosis, as 'living made easy', and dysbiosis as 'difficult living' (Furney, 1891: 11). Other than a further reference to the present age as an 'electrical age' or an 'age of eubiosis' (Furney, 1891: 54), there is not much in the book about the two terms. It is true, however, as Ariel Rawson has noted in her PhD dissertation (2021), that Hooks and O'Malley are a bit too quick to dismiss this source as fictional and hence 'misleading' in the ancestry of contemporary concepts of dysbiosis. As with other science fiction writers at the time, Furney builds on the imaginary of biological plasticity to highlight the technological potential to manipulate life forms in the service of futuristic progress goals (immortality, rejuvenation), often with a racialised overtone. Dysbiosis and eubiosis are, for Furney 'methods of culturing: environmental directions that produce distinct hereditary effects' (Rawson 2021: 179). As Rawson further writes:

> Rather than quickly dismiss the link between eugenic thought and contemporary uses of the concepts dysbiosis and eubiosis as 'dubious' or irrelevant, I take the eugenic connections to dysbiosis-eubiosis as a serious area for interrogation and thus take seriously the potential legacies of Furney's novel too.
>
> *(Rawson, 2021: 179)*

Interestingly, it is to Furney's work that the Planetary Health literature (Logan et al., 2016) refers when looking for the origin of the notion of life in distress.

Rejecting this proto-eugenic matrix is complicated especially for the third author selected by Hook and O'Malley. A prominent chemist and director of the Reichsanstalt für Vitaminprüfung und Vitaminforschung (Reich Institute for Vitamin Testing and Vitamin Research) in Leipzig (1942–1945), and from 1951, Head of the Institute for Nutrition and Dietary Science in what was the then DDR, Scheunert used the term Dybiosis (*Dysbiose der Darmflora*) in 1920, well before he became involved with Nazism and in the context of veterinary not human research on normality and abnormality in the intestine flora of horses. However, he made a link with human research when the political conditions were right. Scheunert investigated the normality and abnormality of human physiological reactions in five experiments carried out between 1938 and 1943 with war and political prisoners (Joost, 2012). As the most prominent German vitamin researcher of his time, he was particularly interested in determining the importance of vitamin A and vitamin B1 requirements and of fortified foods, of which he was a proponent (unlike other Nazi organic food supporters). While the term dysbiosis was not (to my knowledge) used in these experiments they were still aimed at determining the right 'balance' of vitamins for populations deemed worthy of being healthy, such as the German army. Once he got ethical and financial approval for a trial project named 'Vitamin balance' (*Vitaminbilanz*), Scheunert carried out research at the Waldheim prison in Saxony which hosted male and female political prisoners sentenced to prolonged internment as well as on factory workers, including Soviet war prisoners, at the Krupp factories. Whether these experiments of induced starvation caused death or only suffering is still open to debate (Thimme (2012) and Joost (2012), reach different conclusions).

Eubiosis – between Living well and eugenics: Wider context

That it is not possible to disentangle the history of many biological concepts from their wider political context is further evidenced by another family connection in the history of dysbiosis and eubiosis. In the 1920s several publications explicitly use the terms *Eubiosis* and *Eubiótico* including work by J. Fernando Carbonell (d. 1947), a rather obscure but interesting libertarian, naturist and anti-Pasteurian figure within intellectual and social reform groups in South America. Carbonell wrote an anti-vaccination and anti-Pasteurian pamphlet in 1907 and later submitted a petition to the Uruguayan parliament against mandatory anti-smallpox vaccination. Carbonell, also known for his previous work on feminism and naturism in which he ties the feminine role to its maternal function against the pretension of masculine-like emancipation (Carbonell, 1909, Cuadro Cawen, 2016), became in the 1920s the editor of the journal *Natura*: a monthly review for propaganda on natural ways of living and vegetarianism. His combination of naturism, eugenics, hygiene, nutrition and temperance is not uncommon in the complex archipelago of anarchist, 'progressive' and often Lamarckian eugenics at the time (Cleminson 2008, Meloni 2016). Carbonell wrote a book on *El vegetarianismo integral único régimen eubiótico* (Integral vegetarianism as the unique Eubiotic regime) and in 1920 he gave a talk in Montevideo, later published as *Conferencia sobre los fundamentos de la eubiosis* (Carbonell, 1920). This book presents Carbonell as Director of the Institute of Practical Eubiosis ('Eubiosis Practica') and it is interesting to see how he positions himself vis-à-vis the then better-known 'English invention' of Galton's Eugenics. As is frequently the case with eugenicists of the time, the attempt is to supplement attention to good birth, as in Galton and later genetics, with a focus on good living (Eubiosis), and even good death (Euthanasia).

Eubiosis is presented as a process that can cure the 'vices and mistakes' of Human civilisation (Carbonell, 1920: 5). In detail the claim is that 'good living' can implement Naturism within civilisation so as to obtain 'the rehabilitation of [humans] primal symbiotic relationships, with those that have become pathogenic agents' (Carbonell, 1920: 9). Symbiosis as a metaphor is then translated to the political field, such that political malaise and corruption are defined as a loss of symbiosis and that the politicians become 'parasite[s] of the people' (Carbonell, 1920: 13). Eubiotic science is hence portrayed by Carbonell as a vast endeavour aimed at repairing broken symbiotic relationships. Eugenics, as invented by Galton, can then be understood only 'as the first chapter of Eubiosis' (Carbonell, 1920: 16). Similar debates were happening in continental Europe at the time. In 1923, Stan Ruziska, a professor of Hygiene at the Faculty of Medicine in Bratislava (then Czechoslovakia) published in French, *Social Eubiotics* (L'Eubiotique sociale) (Ruziska, 1923). The book has a long but very explicative subtitle: *Family life in close connection with nature is the only possible natural basis for any popular culture – A basis blindly neglected and forgotten by current culture.* As with Carbonell, the emphasis is on the imperative of living naturally (focusing in particular on the familial level) in a modern civilisation that has lost touch with its natural basis (the shock of WWI was just a few years behind). While there is no reference to rewilding or probiotic politics in a contemporary sense, Ruziska suggests that cities should only be used during working hours and that people should live in rural areas, or new built garden cities, where they can re-establish lost connections with natural life. Ruziska's book was reviewed in *The British Medical Journal* (James, 1924) with the reviewer identifying a parallel with eugenics: 'Eubiotics' the reviewer of the brief note writes, 'may be defined as the science of *living a healthy life* just as eugenics may be defined as *the science of producing a healthy life*' (James, 1924: 1119) (my italics).[2] Finally, another contemporary expression of similar ideas is provided by Dr Iago Galdston, a US based psychiatrist who published an article in *Science* titled 'Eubiotic medicine'. To quote:

> I should like to submit the term 'eubiotic medicine 'to take the place of or to supplement the term 'preventive medicine.' I intend this term to indicate those phases of medical science and of medical service *which go beyond the prevention of disease* and which foster as well as advance the biologic growth, development and well-being of the individual.
>
> *(Galdston 1944: 76) (my italics)*

Galdston went on to publish several books in medicine and psychiatry after WWII, in which he used the term 'eubiotic'. For instance, in *The Meaning of Social Medicine*, Galdston writes about the importance of focusing on 'eubiotic medicine', that is 'medicine dedicated to helping the individual *to achieve the best* that he is capable of in his experience in living' (Galdston, 1954: 92) (my italics).

While it is always risky to draw historical analogies, it is interesting to note that this early twentieth century literature relies on a number of tropes that recur in contemporary iterations of dysbiosis and eubiosis, including an emphasis on the damaging effects of industrialised life; a romanticisation of living symbiotically or in harmony with nature; a sense of the plasticity of biological life); and a notion that science could play a positive role in fostering healthier and more vital populations.

Balance, Galenism and the microbiome: A microbiopolitics of temperance avant la lettre

My first and still early genealogy has identified continuities in the use of terms like balance within wider eugenic and biopolitical ideas about life and how it is governed. My next move is to return to the second key point made by O'Malley and colleagues about the surprising symbiosis, or as they write 'uncanny resemblance', between concepts elaborated in Galenism, particularly the notion of balance/imbalance, and contemporary microbiome research. To sum up their most recent claims, Sumrall and O'Malley write:

> both Galenic medicine and medical microbiome research rely heavily on notions of imbalance and balance (….), with *undesirable unbalanced states* called 'dyskrasia' and 'dysbiosis' respectively. Therapeutically, both systems aim at restoration to a balanced state. Both traditions also hold that the composition of the focal entities (humours or microbiomes) determines *not just every bodily state but mental ones too*. Causality for both is conceived teleologically, meaning that parts of bodies 'function for' the maintenance of the whole. And ultimately, each framework asserts that external environments are part of the balance equation, thereby situating the humours or microbiomes in a unified multilevel theory that purportedly explains *the very nature of health and perhaps even humans*.
> (*Sumrall and O'Malley, 2024: 1) (my italics)*

I find this point particularly intriguing in the light of my previous genealogy which ties dysbiosis/eubiosis to biopolitics and eugenics. Indeed, Galenism is another perfect example of biopolitics *avant la lettre*, in that it is impossible to disentangle medical ideas from wider notions of intervention to promote a good or healthy life and amend or condemn unhealthy one. Galenism, an umbrella term here for medical humoralism and its several ramifications in Eurasia including, decisively for Western medicine, medieval Persian-Arabic medicine, is often misleadingly interpreted as a view of medicine unaware of the modern notions of normality and abnormality.

Unfortunately, Foucault (building on Canguilhem) has made this view a cornerstone of his account of the modern birth of biopolitics by claiming famously that 'up to the end of the eighteenth-century medicine related much more to health than to normality' (Foucault, 2002: 35). According to this version, it is only with the modern authoritarian power of medicine that new social demands are attached to medical values and notions of health and illness are turned into technologies of normalisation by a plethora of experts. This interpretation is repeated over and over by Foucauldian scholarship, becoming canonical and largely unproblematised in social studies of health. Recent historiography has challenged this position by showing that humoral medicine was far from being removed from notions of normality and abnormality; that these understandings were applied at the individual and collective level; and that medical, political and religious metaphors were mixed with ideas about the malleability of humours to produce a technology of normalisation and subjectivation (Geltner, 2019).

Humoral medicine even became a source of racial taxonomies based on people's different environmental exposures and on alleged physical/moral qualities at the group level (Weeda, 2021). More broadly, under the influence of humoralism, the whole medieval culture was shaped by an imperative towards balance and the avoidance of imbalance (Kaye, 2014). In politics, theology and natural philosophy, a pervasive language of symmetry, temperance, proportionality and midpoint (*medietas*), became ubiquitous and increasingly sophisticated. For centuries, such Galenic thinking shaped understandings of the body, cities, and political institutions as systems in dynamic equilibrium that can quickly lose their balance and become loaded by humoral excesses.

The normative angle here is difficult to miss and is epitomised by Galen's notions of *eukrasia* (well-proportioned mixing or complexion) and *dyskrasia* (bad mixing). As one can discover in the *Tegni*, the most well-read medieval summary of Galenic medical work in Latin, any deviation of a body 'from its normal nature' (towards the hot and the dry or wet and cold, for instance) must be re-balanced by a medicine 'that is proportional to the magnitude of the ill-balance (*discrasie*) of the complexion' (Kaye, 2014: 163). Similarly, to restore to moderation (*ad moderatum reduci*) what is 'ill-proportioned' (*immoderatum*) and 'contrary to nature' the physician should look for something that is 'equally ill-proportioned in the contrary direction' (Kaye, 2014: 165). With this subtle and dynamic ontology and techniques of balancing and counterbalancing, medical humoralism became the key source of an early modern microbiopolitics based on notions of temperance and prudence, but also aware of the risks of a '*distemperata complexio*'.

Vigilance on the six key elements of a healthy lifestyle (or six Galenic non-naturals: passions, air or climate, food and its method of preparation, repletion and evacuation, sleeping and vigil, and exercise) pushed people to enter a relationship of self- governance and self-examination with their own bodies.[3] The wider religious (Christian or Islamic for instance) context in which this self-refashioning took shape had the further effect of loading medical terminology with moralistic meaning. Galenic biology remained a hopeful one, though: an unbalanced individual constitution could always be turned into a balanced one 'by dint of reason, and a sober life' so as to 'live to a great age and in good health' (Cornaro, 1833: 98). Interestingly, however, this malleability had limits, both individual and collective. In Renaissance versions known as geohumoralism 'regionally framed' version of humoralist ideas were applied to whole groups becoming a key source of early modern racial classifications. In humoralism, the importance of food in establishing and maintaining whole groups' biological identity has been emphasised by scholars, particularly in context of early modern colonialism which could imply a change in diet, waters, or climate for European settlers. Good Spanish food, for instance, would be vital in maintaining or dissolving 'the most fundamental of colonial divisions: that between the bodies of the colonisers and the colonised' (Earle, 2012: 183).

Much earlier than these colonial explorations, and already in Galen's writings (2nd CE), poor food was thought to make people's aspect and physiology so diverse as to become nearly unrecognisable to an expert medical gaze. This is why Galen takes peasants to be an entirely alien species, animals ('donkeys') in their constitution, when compared to the physiological standard shaped by his own experience of being an 'affluent, urban, Greek male, in the prime of life' (Mattern, 2008: 105). This point needs a bit more elaboration.

In the previous section I showed that terms like eubiosis and dysbiosis cannot be disentangled from their wider biopolitical context or from their ties with eugenic ideas and temperance/naturism in the early 20th century. In this section I have suggested that if we take seriously the return to Galenism implicit in the notion of balance and imbalance in microbiome research, as claimed by O'Malley and colleagues, there might be a second genealogical lineage that reinforces the implicit biopolitical meaning of terms like eubiosis and dysbiosis: that is the moralised micropolitics of balance and imbalance linked with Galenic medicine in its different iterations in Eurasia.

In other words, there is not only an epistemological confusion: modern microbiome research does not rely on outdated or circular concepts, rather it imbues them with a set of highly normative assumptions that reinforce moral and social not just medical norms (moderation, vigilance on lifestyle, normality and abnormality). In modern biomedicine, this scrutiny is applied to individuals and to populations at risk of becoming out of balance. In the final part of the chapter, I revisit studies of vulnerable populations and situate these accounts within a broader framework of proto-eugenic notions that have never been properly dispelled by the scientific literature and that are still used, unreflectively, in medical microbiome research.

The burden of plasticity: Life in distress as populations out of balance

Several recent articles have noted the tendency in microbiome research to identify biological groups based on microbiome findings, for instance linking 'groups that are considered to be human races and their health status with geography-specific, nationality-specific, and/or lifestyle-specific variations in microbiomes in the oral cavity, respiratory tract, skin, urogenital tract, and in the digestive system' (Nieves Delgado and Baedke, 2021: 3). Adverse health outcomes and, more broadly, racial differences in health, are often connected to differences in the microbiome, for instance, to infections and the composition of the vaginal microbiome for black and Hispanic women in the US (Benezra, 2020). Similar claims are increasing in epigenomics and in ideas about the Developmental Origins of Health and Disease. In both fields, methods of classifying groups based on DNA methylation (an epigenetic biomarker), encourage essentialist interpretations of acquired differences among ethnic/race based groups related to repeated exposure to specific diets or environments.

With this often comes a tendency to describe minority groups in terms of a damage or deficit narrative that may encourage stigma. Moll et al. (2024) make a similar point, tracking an expansion of neuroscience, epigenetic and developmental plasticity studies in postcolonial settings and noting the use of these concepts, particularly in health economics, to explain differences in health and human capital outcomes among marginalised groups in postcolonial settings. While usually framed in terms of the hopeful image of a window of plasticity that should galvanize investment at the right time (often the first 1,000 days of life, from preconception to year 2), some of this literature generates a darker model of health deficit in which accumulated histories of imbalance cannot be rebalanced.

When used in this way, the concept of a window of plasticity may turn into its opposite – as is the case with evidence that, after a threshold has been passed in human development, some groups are permanently 'scarred'. The claim is that because of the accumulated adverse effects of the biological system's memory, human capital can become too degraded to recover (Moll et al., 2024). In the macro-ecology literature too, the notion of 'hysteresis',[4] that is the overall dependence of a system on its history – from the Greek *husteréō*, 'lagging behind, occurring later' – addresses the cost/efforts or irreversibility of effects in degraded ecologies.

As represented here, the dependence of a system (a forest, an ocean) on its history may prevent or delay restoration or reproduce trajectories that do not follow the original path (Beisner et al., 2003; Staal et al., 2020). After certain tipping points are passed, critical processes may become unavoidably irreversible.

This biology of the aftermath (Landecker, 2024) is particularly evident in studies of human populations exposed to extremely degrading events such as ethnic cleansing, war, famine or forced displacement. At a time of genocidal violence and forced human migration as a result of ecological or political changes, emerging sciences in postgenomics have started to document the impact of this violence on the bodies of vulnerable groups. Studies of epigenetic signatures as well as telomere length, and allostatic and inflammation loads in vulnerable populations have documented the molecular underpinning of adverse events and the development of resilience, particularly in children (Kertes et al., 2016; Serpeloni et al., 2019; Merrill et al., 2025).[5]

The frequent recourse to a terminology of load and overload in this literature is something that needs some consideration given that metaphors in science are never neutral and that they are reflexively or unreflexively used to convey specific meanings often reproducing existing social norms and values in how natural entities are framed. In this context, it is important to notice that studies of the microbiome of refugee populations have started to appear at a growing rate in the scientific literature, documenting imbalances in the gut microbiome and their relationship to mental health conditions among refugees and asylum seekers (Comelli et al., 2024). More specifically, Palladino et al. (2025) have recently conducted a one-year study of the gut microbiome composition of newly arrived African asylum seekers in Italy, comparing them to traditional rural populations from the country of origin and noting the loss of microbial diversity as an emerging biomarker of stress and trauma with important implications for health and targeted medical intervention. Similarly, Shahzad and colleagues (2025) assessed gut-microbiome diversity and associated demographic and nutritional factors in a cohort of more than 200 adolescent Afghans in the Khazana refugee camp (Peshawar) in Pakistan. This study shows that normal-weight adolescents host a more diverse microbiome compared to the undernourished group and looks with optimism to Vitamin D supplements as a means of modifying gut microbiota composition.

The article by Shazad et al. emphasises the restorative side of food intervention, hence the claim that 'Nutritional status *reshapes* gut microbiota composition in adolescent Afghan refugees' (Shahzad et al., 2025). These, and other studies looking at 'holistic approaches for improving the health of such understudied and vulnerable populations' (Shahzad et al., 2025: 65) can be seen as part of a 'humanitarian biomedicine' logic that that can sustain more discriminatory arguments (Lakoff, 2010). This is the case, for instance, in a 2016 German study of the resistome of refugees from Syria, Iraq and Afghanistan in Germany that, 'for the first time, assess[ed] antibiotic resistance genes in refugees and demonstrate[d] a substantially increased prevalence for most resistances compared to German controls' (Häsler et al, 2018: 1).

Next, there is repeated reference to a second type of imbalance, namely the economic burden of dealing with 'the antibiotic resistome in refugees':

> infections caused by these pathogens are associated with increased mortality, duration of hospital stay, and hospital costs *with large economic impact* on public health systems (Häsler et al., 2018: 1) (my italics). See also Reinheimer et al., 2016, and for social commentary Kamenshchikova et al., 2023.

The article by Häsler et al. ends on the note that:

> the potential consequences for healthcare systems of host countries warrant a careful and systematic evaluation of the natural course and impact of resistomes in the clinical and outpatient setting.
>
> *(Häsler et al., 2018: 9)*

This oscillation between 'malleability' or restoration and 'essentialism' that fixes whole populations to a biological discourse of risk and acquired damage has been tracked in epigenetic research (Warin et al., 2020; Keaney et al., 2024). Microbiome studies of vulnerable populations seem to follow a similar logic. This movement between hopeful and 'destructive plasticity' (Malabou, 2012; Du Plessis, 2023) seems inherent to postgenomic discourses that rely on notions of the epigenome or the microbiome as plastic and hence amenable to intervention but also sculpted by life events beyond control of the individual.[6] This is exactly the point when plasticity turns from hope into a *burden*, a stigma associated with risky or difficult populations too damaged or infectious to be treatable within the 'reasonable' limits assigned to the health or political system.

This representation, with its uneven geography of risk and threat, is particularly visible in accounts of the spread of AMR and of how this is connected to international travels, forced migrations, and armed conflicts. More abstractly, it is part of a longer history of foreign microbial threat, border crossing, and imperial hygiene (Kraut, 1995; Bashford, 2003). However, the way in which postgenomic and wider biomedical debates blur the line between what is fixed at birth (hereditary) and what is acquired from recent life events, indicates the confluence of other, less visible lines of protoeugenic thinking in the 20th century.

A case in point is the now nearly forgotten debate on 'genetic load', the tendency, hypothesised by Nobel Laureate, geneticist and eugenicist H. J. Muller (1950), for deleterious mutations to accumulate in specific populations due, for instance, to exposure to radiation (Paul, 1987). A darker version of the term *load* can be found in the history of early 20th century German psychiatry first, and Nazi eugenics later, with the notion of *Belastung* (strain, load, burden) often associated to the adjective *erblich* (hereditary) to refer to mentally ill individuals (Teicher, 2018). These and other eugenic references are extreme but they suggest that modern attempts to optimise life (eu-genics) are always on the verge of turning into a discourse of less optimal or less capable bodies and minds (according to this prototype), that is, into dysgenic forms of life that represent a burden on human society.

The vision of dysgenic life was a key biopolitical figure in intra-war biology, being embraced by both hard hereditarians geneticists and Lamarckians, right and leftwing alike, and used to denounce the degenerative effects of modern civilisation (see Meloni (2016) for an analysis). Although notions like epigenetic or dysbiotic load are mobilised today, they are so sparsely and in ways that are entirely removed from eugenic implications in a 20th century sense.

Despite their strongly normative meaning of good or failed living, concepts of eubiosis and dysbiosis are currently operationalised in ways that do not make further assumptions about who is or is not worthy of living, or that imply a larger agenda – for example, to fight the 'vices and mistake' of our civilisation in the sense that Carbonell described in the early 1920s.

Nonetheless, a word of caution is in order. Eugenics never existed in a singular form, nor was it ever the result of an accumulation of scientific evidence. It was instead the sudden outcome of rapidly mutated political circumstances that made possible what was unthinkable until just a few years before (Meloni, 2016). The Foucauldian biopolitics of life and biomedicine in the early 21st century has tended to downplay the risk of eugenics and has instead focused on narratives of individual freedom, the power of experts, subjectivity and emerging forms of biocitisenship (Rose, 2007). However, the unequal experience of COVID-19 has shown that for a significant part of the world's population, a post-disciplinary power of care is not the main framework through which people experience life and death. Instead, the experience is of the exact opposite: a governmentality through inaction, distrust of expertise, data poverty, and failure, on the part of the state, to protect lives from imminent danger (Meloni and Vatter, 2023).

More abstractly, epigenomic and microbiome medical studies are turning their attention to calamitous events, and to the possibility of ontological annihilation for humans living in extremely degraded circumstances (Du Plessis, 2023; Malabou 2012). This interest is the end-product of structural violence and ecological degradation and displacement (Aggarwal and Aggarwal, 2025), coexisting with, and alongside, liberal, post-liberal, and non-liberal forms of governmentality.

In accounting for the biological signatures of dysbiotic life, human and more-than-human, emerging sciences like microbiome medicine and epigenetics have a responsibility to do that in a way that does not harm and that possibly empowers injured lives and living. As other chapters in this book show, one way of fostering this awareness is to keep a plurality of disciplinary perspectives in view. This helps avoid the simplifying effects of microbial narratives that are disentangled from wider socioeconomic and structural inequalities. As the editors of this book point out in their introduction, the challenge is to avoid positions that are 'too stable, abstract, partial or siloed' and that are 'therefore incapable of addressing global challenges ahead'.

In conclusion, the politics of knowledge of concepts now used in microbiome and medicine, and the weight of their accumulated history, needs to be recognised if we are to acknowledge the societal inequalities and structural violence inscribed in the unbalanced or distressed bodies of specific groups or populations (Warin et al., 2011). As with other areas of postgenomics, microbiome research can be developed and positioned within different and often competing ontologies and political agendas. If anything, this makes it even more important to be aware of long-standing cultural templates that might unwittingly shape the way we think about life and death, health and disease. This nexus between the politics of knowledge and scientific language is unavoidable in the history of science; it is even less avoidable in emerging and still relatively unformed disciplines like microbiome research, especially when those fields address vulnerable human groups, and take place in an epistemically unjust global health field (Bhakuni and Abimbola, 2021)

Notes

1 A number of -omics disciplines like epigenomics, microbiomics and exposomics that have emerged after the deciphering of the HGP in 2003 and lead to a wider reconsideration of environmental factors in the causation and origin of disease and development.
2 The adjective *eubiotique* is already attested in Littré's *Dictionnaire de la langue française* (1877) as a 'philosophical term' indicating 'the set of principles relatives to the art of good living' (*bien vivre*). Littré was also the French translator of all Hippocrates corpus: this entry may somehow indicate a reference to works in the area of Hippocratic–Galenic conduct for a healthy living.
3 This section sums up Chapter 2 of my book *Impressionable Biologies* (Routledge, 2019). A broader literature on these influences on a pre- and early modern biopolitics can be found there.
4 I thank Jamie Lorimer for calling my attention to this aspect.
5 I thank Natasha Rooney for her initial research in this area.
6 Interestingly, microbiome research, as epigenetics does, is also increasingly looking at the first thousand days of life (from conception to year 2) as the period of 'establishment' of the gut microbiota of the child with long-lasting consequences on disease risk in adult life (Rautava, 2016). Notions of 'early programming' seem to be shared by both fields (Indrio et al., 2017).

References

Aggarwal, S., and Aggarwal, P. (2025). 'Ecological displacement and structural injustice: rethinking protection in a collapsing world', *Journal of Global Ethics*, 21(1): 77–84. https://doi.org/10.1080/17449626.2025.2503878.

Bashford, A. (2003). *Imperial Hygiene: A critical history of colonialism, nationalism and public health*. London: Palgrave Macmillan.

Beisner, B. E., Haydon, D. T., and Cuddington, K. (2003). 'Alternative stable states in ecology', *Frontiers in Ecology and the Environment*, 1(7): 376–382. https://doi.org/10.1890/1540-9295(2003)001[0376:ASSIE]2.0.CO;2.

Benezra, A. (2020). 'Race in the microbiome', *Science, Technology and Human Values*, 45(5): 877–902. https://doi.org/10.1177/0162243920911998.

Bhakuni, H., & Abimbola, S. (2021). Epistemic injustice in academic global health. The Lancet Global Health, 9(10), e1465-e1470.

Brüssow, H. (2020). 'Problems with the concept of gut microbiota dysbiosis', *Microbial Biotechnology*, 13: 423–434. https://doi.org/10.1111/1751-7915.13479.

Carbonell, J. F. (1909). *Feminismo y Marimachismo*. Montevideo: Centro Natura.

Carbonell, J. F. (1920). *Conferencia Sobre los Fundamentos de la Eubiosis*. Habana: Imprenta Molina.

Cleminson, R. (2008). *Anarquismo y Sexualidad en España, 1900-1939*. Cadiz: Servicio Publicaciones UCA.

Comelli, A., Gaviraghi, A., Cattaneo, P., Motta, L., Bisoffi, Z., and Stroffolini, G. (2024). 'Antimicrobial resistance in migratory paths, refugees, asylum seekers and internally displaced persons: A narrative review', *Current Tropical Medicine Reports*, 11(3): 153–166.
Cornaro, L. (1833). *Sure and Certain Methods of Attaining a Long and Healthful Life*. Cheltenham: GA Williams (trans.).
Cuadro Cawen, I. (2016). *Feminismos, culturas políticas e identidades de género en Uruguay (1906-1932)*. PhD Dissertation: University of Sevilla.
Du Plessis, G. (2023). 'Destructive plasticity and the microbial geopolitics of childhood malnutrition', *Review of International Studies*, 49(2): 300–318. https://doi.org/10.1017/S0260210522000328.
Earle, R. (2012). *The Body of the Conquistador*. Cambridge: Cambridge University Press.
Foucault, M. (2002). *The Birth of the Clinic*. London: Routledge.
Furney, E. E. (1891). *Culture, a modern method*. New York/St Louis: I.H. Brown and Company.
Galdston, I. (1944). 'Eubiotic medicine', *Science*, 100(2587): 74–76.
Galdston, I. (1954). *The Meaning of Social Medicine*. New York: Commonwealth Fund.
Geltner, G. (2019). *Roads to Health: Infrastructure and urban wellbeing in later medieval Italy*. Philadelphia: University of Pennsylvania Press.
Häsler, R., Kautz, C., Rehman, A., Podschun, R., Gassling, V., Brzoska, P. and Schreiber, S. (2018). 'The antibiotic resistome and microbiota landscape of refugees from Syria, Iraq and Afghanistan in Germany', *Microbiome*, 6(1): 37. https://doi.org/10.1186/s40168-018-0414-7.
Hooks, K. B., and O'Malley, M. A. (2017). 'Dysbiosis and its discontents', *mBio*, 8, e01492–17. https://doi.org/10.1128/mbio.01492-17.
Indrio, F., Martini, S., Francavilla, R., Corvaglia, L., Cristofori, F., Mastrolia, S. A., and Loverro, G. (2017). 'Epigenetic matters: the link between early nutrition, microbiome, and long-term health development', *Frontiers in pediatrics, 5*, 178. https://doi.org/10.3389/fped.2017.00178.
James, C. (1924). 'Eubiotics'. *British Medical Journal*. Dec 13: 1119–1120.
Joost, H. G. (2012). 'Carl Arthur Scheunert's experiments on human nutrition, 1938-1943: boundary transgressions of a scientist under national socialism', *Medizinhistorisches Journal*, 47(4): 296–334.
Kamenshchikova, A., Wolffs, P. F., Hoebe, C. J., Penders, J. and Horstman, K. (2023). 'Metaphors of foreign strangers: antimicrobial resistance in biomedical discourses', *Science as Culture*, 32(2): 294–314. https://doi.org/10.1080/09505431.2023.2180628.
Kaye, J. A. (2014). *History of Balance, 1250–1375: The emergence of a new model of equilibrium and its impact on thought*. Cambridge: Cambridge University Press.
Keaney, J., Byrne, H., Warin, M. and Kowal, E. (2024). 'Intergenerational Trauma' in Pentecost, M., Keaney, J., Moll, T. and Penkler, M. (eds.) *The handbook of DOHaD and society*, 166–173.
Kertes, D. A., Kamin, H. S., Hughes, D. A., Rodney, N. C., Bhatt, S., and Mulligan, C. J. (2016). 'Prenatal Maternal Stress Predicts Methylation of Genes Regulating the Hypothalamic–Pituitary–Adrenocortical System in Mothers and Newborns in the Democratic Republic of Congo', *Child Development*, 87(1): 61–72. https://doi.org/10.1111/cdev.12487.

Kim, B.S., Jeon, Y.S. and Chun J. (2013). 'Current status and future promise of the human microbiome', *Pediatr Gastroenterol Hepatol Nutr,* 16: 71–79. https://doi.org/10.5223/pghn.2013.16.2.71.

Kraut, A. M. (1995). *Silent Travellers: Germs, genes, and the immigrant menace.* Baltimore: Johns Hopkins University Press.

Lakoff, A. (2010). 'Two regimes of global health', *Humanity: An International Journal of Human Rights, Humanitarianism, and Development, 1*(1): 59–79.

Landecker, H. (2024). 'Life as Aftermath: Social Theory for an Age of Anthropogenic Biology', *Science, Technology and Human Values,* 5(4):697–712. https://doi.org/10.1177/01622439241233946.

Logan, A.C., Jacka, F.N., and Prescott, S.L. (2016). 'Immune-Microbiota Interactions: Dysbiosis as a Global Health Issue', *Curr. Allergy Asthma Rep*, 1–9. https://doi.org/10.1007/s11882-015-0590-5.

Malabou, C. (2012). *Ontology of the Accident: An essay on destructive plasticity.* Oxford: Polity Press.

Mattern, S. P. (2008). *Galen and the Rhetoric of Healing.* Baltimore: Johns Hopkins University Press.

Meloni, M. (2016). *Political Biology: Science and social values in human heredity from eugenics to epigenetics.* Basingstoke: Palgrave Macmillan. https://doi.org/10.1057/9781137377722.

Meloni, M. (2019). *Impressionable Biologies: From the archaeology of plasticity to the sociology of epigenetics.* London: Routledge. https://doi.org/10.4324/9781315169583.

Meloni, M., and Vatter, M. (2023). 'Biopolitics after COVID: Notes from the Crisis', *Theory and Event*, 26(2): 368–392.

Merrill, S. M., Konwar, C., Fraihat, Z., Parent, J. and Dajani, R. (2025). 'Molecular insights into trauma: A framework of epigenetic pathways to resilience through intervention', *Med*, 6(2). https://doi.org/10.1016/j.medj.2024.11.013.

Moll, T., Meloni, M., and Issaka, A. (2024). 'Foetal programming meets human capital: biological plasticity, development, and the limits to the economization of life', *BioSocieties*, 19(3): 424–451. https://doi.org/10.1057/s41292-023-00309-8.

Nag, S., Srivastava, N., Dutta, R., Bagchi, A., Adur, I. and Chakraborty, S. (2023). 'Connection between Dysbiosis and Diet' in Srivastava, N. Ibrahim, S., Chattopadhyay, J. and Arbab, M. (eds). *The Gut Microbiota in Health and Disease*, Oxford: Wiley. 55–79.

Nieves Delgado, A., and Baedke, J. 2021. 'Does the human microbiome tell us something about race?', *Humanities and Social Sciences Communications*, 8(1): 1–12. https://doi.org/10.1057/s41599-021-00772-3.

O'Malley, M. A. (2024). 'The concept of balance in microbiome research', *Bioessays*, 46(8): 2400050. https://doi.org/10.1002/bies.202400050.

Paasch, B. C., Sohrabi, R., Kremer, J. M., Nomura, K., Cheng, Y. T., Martz, J. and He, S. Y. (2023). 'A critical role of a eubiotic microbiota in gating proper immunocompetence in Arabidopsis', *Nature Plants*, 9(9): 1468–1480. https://doi.org/10.1038/s41477-023-01501-1.

Palladino, G., Marangi, M., Scicchitano, D., Turroni, S., Rampelli, S. and Candela, M. (2025). 'Gut microbiome structure in asylum seekers newly arrived in Italy from Africa', *Sci Rep*, 15(1): 40596. https://doi.org/10.1038/s41598-025-24250-x.

Paul, D. B. (1987). '"Our Load of Mutations" Revisited', *Journal of the History of Biology,* 321–335.

Rautava, S. (2016). 'Early microbial contact, the breast milk microbiome and child health', *Journal of developmental origins of health and disease*, 7(1): 5–14. https://doi.org/10.1017/S2040174415001233.

Rawson, A. (2021). *Black fungibility and the PosthuMan: Becoming microbial geographies*. Doctoral Dissertation. Ohio State University.

Reinheimer, C., Kempf, V.A.J., Gottig, S., Hogardt, M., Wichelhaus, T.A., O'Rourke, F. and Brandt, C., (2016). 'Multidrug-resistant organisms detected in refugee patients admitted to a University Hospital, Germany June-December 2015', *Euro Surveill*, 21(2): 1–5. https://doi.org/10.2807/1560-7917.es.2016.21.2.30110.

Rose, N. (2007). *The politics of life itself*. Princeton: Princeton University Press.

Ruziska, S. (1923). *L'Eubiotique sociale*. Paris: A. Maloine et Fils.

Scheunert, C. A. (1920). ŭber Knowchenweiche bei Pferden und 'Dysbiose der Darmflora'. Zeitschrift fŭr Infektionskrankheiten, XXI: 105–120.

Shahzad, M., Arshad, M., Ahmad, H.A., Iddrissu, I., Bailey, E.H., Dru, N., Khan, S., Khan, H. and Andrews, S.C. (2025). 'Nutritional status reshapes gut microbiota composition in adolescent Afghan refugees in Peshawar, Pakistan', *Nutrition Research*, 138: 55–67. https://doi.org/10.1016/j.nutres.2025.04.004.

Staal, A., Fetzer, I., Wang-Erlandsson, L., Bosmans, J. H., Dekker, S. C., van Nes, E. H. and Tuinenburg, O. A. (2020). 'Hysteresis of tropical forests in the 21st century', *Nature communications*, *11*(1): 4978. https://doi.org/10.1038/s41467-020-18728-7.

Sumrall, L. and O'Malley, M. A. (2024). 'Conceptual parallels: Microbiome research and ancient medicine', *Perspectives in Biology and Medicine*, 67(3): 406–423. https://doi.org/10.1353/pbm.2024.a936218.

Teicher, A. (2018). Caution, overload: The troubled past of genetic load, *Genetics*, 210(3), 747–755.

Thimme, R. (2012). 'Carl Arthur Scheunert. Ein Naturwissenschaftler im nationalsozialistischen und im real-sozialistischen Herrschaftssystem', *Zeitschrift für Geschichtswissenschaft*, 60: 5–27.

Warin, M., Kowal, E., and Meloni, M. (2020). 'Indigenous knowledge in a postgenomic landscape: The politics of epigenetic hope and reparation in Australia', *Science, Technology and Human Values*, *45*(1): 87–111. https://doi.org/10.1177/0162243919831077.

Warin, M., Moore, V., Zivkovic, T. and Davies, M. (2011). 'Telescoping the origins of obesity to women's bodies: How gender inequalities are being squeezed out of Barker's hypothesis', *Annals of Human Biology*, *38*(4): 453–460. https://doi.org/10.3109/03014460.2011.591829.

Weeda, C. (2021). *Ethnicity in medieval Europe, 950-1250: Medicine, power and religion*. Woodbridge: Boydell and Brewer.

11

EPIDEMIOLOGY, INDIVIDUALISM AND THE VIRUS

A critical analysis of policy responses to COVID-19 in the UK

Michael P. Kelly and Elizabeth Shove

Introduction

In this chapter we focus on specific aspects of the COVID-19 pandemic in the UK, and the government's response to this unprecedented public health emergency. As we explain, interventions and policies relied on particular forms of scientific thinking, notably epidemiological modelling and virological aetiology (Horton, 2020), and a raft of related assumptions about individual behaviour, pathways of infection and the independence of coexisting conditions and diseases. This brought with it increased rather than decreased risk from the virus.

The COVID-19 pandemic created medical, political, ideological and scientific problems for governments, medical authorities and international agencies. The pandemic led to the deaths of at least three million people globally and more than 225,000 in the UK (Hallett, 2024). Public health authorities worldwide had anticipated a global pandemic for many decades. Pandemics occur cyclically and although there had been examples of major outbreaks of infectious disease, notably various influenza epidemics, there had not been a truly global pandemic since the Spanish Flu of 1918 (Hallett, 2024). Unsurprisingly, there were different degrees of preparedness. Some jurisdictions were considered to be in a much better position than others and the UK was one of several countries that had detailed plans in place. As events unfolded, the plans that had been designed in the expectation of an influenza pandemic (Department of Health, 2011), proved to be wide of the mark. It was not of course only Britain that got it wrong. The response globally was less than optimal.

DOI: 10.4324/9781003685210-15

COVID-19 was declared a Public Health Emergency of International Concern (PHEIC) on 30 January 2020. The World Health Organisation and nations across the globe responded, though with different degrees of urgency, detail and emphasis. In the UK, government strategies were based on three taken-for-granted assumptions, the apparent self-evidence of which was largely unchallenged.

The first assumption was of the primacy of the acting, self-directed individual human agent. Self-directed agency and therefore responsibility and accountability are deeply sedimented in Western societies and in Britain in particular – in law, in accounts of human actions, and, importantly in this context, in interpretations of medical and psychological science. One part of this is the idea that individual humans are bounded biologically by the skin of the human body and are therefore separate from the environments they inhabit and from other humans. In what has often been called the medical model (Laing, 1976), the locus of understanding disease, including COVID-19, how the virus infected people, how it made them sick and how it killed them, is the individual human body. What individuals do or did to make themselves vulnerable to infection, or to protect themselves from the virus was consequently framed as a matter of personal conduct and responsibility. From this point of view, the social environments in which people live and work, and those individuals' life histories provide either background and context for what is going on, and/or constitute the pool of potential risks like viruses, bacteria, toxins and accidents, which invade or strike the individual with pathological consequences.

The second assumption had to do with the expected form of transmission. In the case of COVID-19, past experiences with influenza were the first point of reference, informing a programme of measures and responses rooted in what proved to be a mistaken or at least partial theory of contagion based on the spread of droplets rather than more diffuse and far-reaching aerosols.

A third related assumption was that the virus was independent, meaning that it was viewed as a material thing in itself, having a biological boundedness (corresponding to what the microorganism looks like under a microscope, and to its microbiological and genomic structure), and being separate from other phenomena in the environmental and ecological world. In essence this led to an emphasis on the modelling the spread of the virus, rather its effects on human health.

This is not to say that biomedical science subscribes to these positions: biomedicine is a great deal more sophisticated than this, and the porousness of the human body and the cells within it are *sine qua non* of medical practice and medical science. But it is to say that in Britain, policy responses and the politics and narratives surrounding the pandemic were dominated by these assumptions. The individualism, whether of persons or viruses, meant that the interrelatedness of people and things as well as microbiological phenomena was set aside, as measures to deal with the infection were put in place. In effect, the measures that were enacted to protect the population from exposure were led by a narrow version of the medical model; by a specific theory of contagion, and by a widely shared view of COVID-19 as an isolated virus, the effects of which were independent from a host of co-existing conditions, co-morbidities and social inequalities. This had profound epistemic consequences in that it led to the side-lining of paradigms, world views and forms of evidence which did not fit with these assumptions. In short, policy responses were informed by a narrow set of ideas about how the virus spreads, not about differential impacts on health and not about the varied conditions and circumstances in which transmission occurred.

In the next section we go into more detail about what happened in the UK before moving on to a review of the social theoretical positions inscribed in policy responses up to and including the programme of mass vaccination.

Responses in the UK

The COVID-19 outbreak began in China in late 2019, and even though this was reported in the broadcast media in the UK, it was just before the Christmas holiday. The outbreak of a pneumonia-type illness in China attracted little attention and most of the British population spent Christmas and New Year largely untroubled by events in a faraway place few people had probably ever heard of. Early into the New Year however, there was greater media coverage of the emerging outbreak and its spread, but in the first few weeks of 2020 the general public did not engage, nor did the NHS (Kelly, 2021). Hospitals continued to function normally and there were no special precautions in place there, or anywhere else. There were no dire warnings from the Department of Health and Social Care or leading politicians in any of the four home countries (England, Wales, Scotland and Northern Ireland), and life carried on pretty much as normal.

As stories of the scale of the crisis began to emerge, especially from Italy, the public did begin to take note, watching in growing horror and disbelief as the Italian health system – which was comparable to that of the UK – was overwhelmed. Although the UK government continued its taciturn *modus operandi*, some event organisers around the country had begun to cancel gatherings, large and small, as they made lay assessments of risk. The government issued advice about protective measures, for example about handwashing, but the strategy that initially dominated in policy and in the English public health agency (Public Health England) was to stop people panicking and to play down the seriousness of what was going on. But of course, the news from around the world was increasingly alarming and a rising number of deaths began to be reported in the British press. Eventually on 23 March 2020, the Prime Minister announced a lockdown. Workplaces, schools, Universities, social events large and small, shops, pubs, restaurants, cafes, were to be closed, and people were told to stay home and avoid social contact where possible.

When the virus first came to light, and in so far as countries were prepared, the working assumption was that the pandemic would be an influenza-type infection and spread in the way influenzas are known to do, with children and schools being crucial for patterns of contagion and with droplets caused by coughing and sneezing being the principal mode of transmission. However, COVID-19 was not an influenza virus, it was a coronavirus. Initially its mode of spread and infectiveness were not understood very well, if at all: for example, it took time to establish that asymptomatic persons who were not coughing and sneezing, could transmit the infection.

To begin with, expected forms of transmission and policies to contain the virus were based on previous experience with influenza. In the UK, the 2011 Strategy about pandemic preparedness specified, amongst other things, surveillance and modelling to detect and assess the impact of any new influenza virus; identification and quantification of the groups most at risk of severe illness, hospitalisation and death; reducing the risk of transmission – through good infection prevention and control practices, for example hand and respiratory hygiene advice (Department of Health, 2011). In the event the modelling did take place along with recommendations about hand hygiene, but as we show below it was seriously deficient in the identification of the groups most likely to suffer the greatest harm.

The first responses were not only driven by a view that the threat was flu-like, but also by the view that everyone was equally at risk, and that whatever measures were to be deployed should be universal ones. In the face of a rapidly spreading novel virus, this was not an unreasonable starting point. Subsequently, data on the differential death rates in different sections of the population has called this assumption into question, but at the time the mantra was one of universal risk.

Through to the end of March into the Spring of 2020 the UK government issued increasingly threatening warnings about the dangers of social contact, and about the risks to everyone, and especially to the NHS. The dangers associated with the disease were extensively publicised and normal life was shut down. People were encouraged to make use of digital technologies for work, for education, and for online shopping. In taking these unprecedented steps, the governments of the four home countries (England, Wales, Scotland and Northern Ireland) repeatedly emphasised the importance of following scientific evidence. But what kind of science?

Following the science: Individualism, transmission and independence

Behind the scenes, and in the face of massive uncertainty, guidance from the UK government was based on scientific evidence grounded in epidemiological modelling and virology, and founded on the three assumptions mentioned above, namely, the importance of individual behaviour, influenza as the reference point for ideas about transmission and contagion, and a view of coronavirus as an independent threat, considered aside from pre- or co-existing conditions, and aside from well-known patterns of health inequality.

The early models (Kucharski et al., 2020) were projections about incidence and were extrapolations based on very limited data, initially from China. As the volume of data grew, models of the 'R' factor, that is the rate at which the virus reproduced, became more sophisticated, but they still assumed a largely homogeneous population with similar patterns of behaviour. They also concentrated on the virus as such, not on the embodied histories of practices and certainly not on the impact of these arrangements on the risks and health effects of infection.

In describing the place of modelling in times of crisis, Anderson (2021) argues that methods of understanding the spread of COVID-19 in the UK resorted to stripped down techniques founded on clearly questionable assumptions about uniform patterns of contamination and contact. As Anderson confirms, these strategies, often based on models of animal disease, took little or no account of sociological understandings of settings and conditions of interaction in the real world. As a result, the idea that populations are heterogeneous and that people's actions and activities within them vary greatly, did not figure in the early modelling scenarios. This was matched by reliance on an also limited body of expertise, despite the existence of much more subtle accounts of disease ecologies and despite the potentially valuable contributions of social research and decades of public health knowledge, experience and practice. Instead, and as Anderson observes, the result was a raft of generic policy measures that tacitly reproduced Margaret Thatcher's famous conclusion that 'there is no such thing as society', and a correspondingly narrow view of 'the virus' and how it spread.

Individual behaviour

Very obviously, actions like eating, shopping, family socialising, the ability to work from home, not to mention skills in digital connectivity or the physical dimensions of indoor and outdoor spaces, are not the same for everyone. However, the fact that the social practices that were potentially relevant for catching or spreading COVID19 differed widely, or that they were very unevenly distributed was routinely overlooked by model builders and policy makers in the UK. Much of the time government advice essentially told people – all people – to do things that mostly they had not done before, had no or little competence or supportive technical infrastructure to do, and that were for some, devoid of meaning. For example, to encourage families to home educate, to tell them not to see their friends and family, to limit the number of times people could leave their homes, to restrict their daily trips to the few shops that were open, or to suggest that the home should become a bounded quarantined environment, was to upend the routine everyday activities and practices of millions of citizens.

What was missing in all this guidance was any serious advice or help about *how* these things might be accomplished. Essentially members of the public were left to work that out for themselves. At the same time to largely ignore the fact that some jobs simply cannot be done online, that many of these involve face to face contact, that some homes are just too small to accommodate every family member in a socially isolated way, and above all that there was a very strong social class gradient in all of this, was to ignore some very basic facts of social, domestic and economic life, not to mention decades of research about these matters.

Anderson suggests that nuanced biosocial understandings (which clearly existed), along with concerns about the importance of social activity, and the 'tangled web of interconnectivity that we call society' (Anderson, 2021:173) were marginalised by an obsession with measurable indicators, including the R 'factor', mentioned above. In his view, the UK government's approach represents a form of biopolitics, and a set of responses that were legitimised in terms of urgency and speed, and that carried with them a host of necessarily invisible social, cultural, political and economic assumptions and priorities.

To reiterate, the government relied on a limited range of theory and evidence, favouring epidemiological analyses grounded in models of atomised, bounded humans interacting in predictable ways (at least predictable in terms of the models). Elaboration of the mechanisms operating in such interactions and any broader conception of linkages and mechanisms between population and outcomes was absent (Russo and Kelly, 2023). In our view, it is naïve and ignorant to think about population-wide interventions without acknowledging the rich heterogeneity and the dynamic nature of populations both in terms of the differential risks of exposure and in terms of the health effects that might follow. Epidemiologists may well respond that they routinely collect data about age, occupation, gender and social differences within populations. This is often so, but our point is that these features are treated as characteristics of individuals, usually analysed cross sectionally at moments in time. Even where longitudinal data are analysed, the characteristics of individuals remain precisely that and they are not conceptualised as dynamic processes or as outcomes or traces of practices, histories and different circumstances (Shove et al., 2026).

Further, the working assumption is that where associations are found between the characteristics about which epidemiology collects data (age, occupation, gender etc.) and various outcomes, the mechanisms involved are similar or the same for everyone (Kelly and Russo, 2021; Russo and Williamson, 2007; 2011). The 'other things being equal' principle of a flat unvariegated social world, effectively rules out systemic understanding of dynamic differences including those of class, gender and ethnicity, ignores the role of institutions and organisations and has only limited connection with the real world. Of course, the old axiom that all models are flawed, but some are useful (Box, 1979), holds, and it would be clearly absurd to dismiss the knowledge gained by and through epidemiology. But the strengths of this sort of science depends on its selective and partial analytic character. And in this case that partiality is also a weakness. The error in policy terms was to treat the bounded nature of epidemiological research as the beginning and the end of the matter, and to fall for a decidedly one-sided view of science and evidence.

There were multiple other approaches – syndemic, complex, sophisticated – that were not given airtime. This is in part about the fashion in ideas, but it is also symptomatic of a trend in policy response and thinking, and of a focus on simple, tractable actionable steps at the cost of all else. It is a classic example of what Daniel Kahneman called fast thinking – i.e. finding quick and simple solutions to complex problems (Kahneman, 2011). Despite and perhaps because of its narrow focus, epidemiological modelling promised to be reliable and defensible 'science', providing a 'safe' point of reference in times of great uncertainty.

Although the range of experts drafted into policy advisory bodies on matters of 'human behaviour' was quite broad, the remit was tightly defined. Social scientists were expected to provide advice on the likely 'public acceptance' of proposed measures. This helps explain the dominance of the Behavioural Insights tradition, and the perceived importance of understanding individual responses to social, economic and environmental cues (Marteau et al., 2011). It also helps explain why information about social heterogeneity was ignored in models of transmission and in the policy actions they informed (Marres and Valderrama Barragán, 2025).

Instead, epidemiological modelling and compatible forms of behavioural research combined to support policy responses that included draconian messaging backed up by legal sanctions for those who failed to comply with rules about social distancing. During the first year of COVID-19 there was a marked shift towards a punishment-centred approach. As the then Secretary of State for Health allegedly put it, let's 'frighten the pants off everyone' (www.bbc.co.uk/news/uk-64848106; Kelly, 2021:321-27). Previous lessons about health and behaviour were side-lined in favour of top-down methods of getting people to comply with directives including methods that had a proven track record of failure (Kelly and Barker, 2016).

The epistemic narrowness of what counted as evidence, the dominance of certain disciplinary perspectives and an unwillingness to engage with wider issues and practices is illustrated by the approach taken by many authorities (including in the UK) to the aetiology of COVID-19 and particularly to its mode of transmission.

Transmission: Droplets and aerosols

There was and still is a difference of scientific opinion about the role of droplets or of aerosols in the spread of COVID-19, and thus about the sort of preventive actions that ought to be promoted. These debates revolve around the process of contagion: does the virus travel by means of droplets emitted during coughing and sneezing or is it airborne, and a consequence of breathing and talking? It has been argued that at the start of the pandemic the dominant view among those advising the UK government, and more broadly, was that the principal mode of transmission was via droplets. This assumption was promulgated by some Infection Control Specialists, and it had profound consequences for narratives about aetiology and spread (Greenhalgh et al., 2024).

The droplet hypothesis is based on the idea that infectious materials (in this case pathogenic particles) are propelled by sneezes and coughing and will travel a relatively short distance (about 2 meters). Because of their mass and gravitation, droplets soon fall to the ground or deposit themselves on surfaces. Social distancing of more than two meters, hand washing and cleaning surfaces are thus the principal means of preventing spread.

The idea of airborne transmission is different. It posits that the infective agent is carried in aerosols and travels much further than 2 meters. Therefore, an important means of preventing the spread of infection will be the wearing of masks and making indoor air quality as good as possible. Greenhalgh and colleagues argue that there is, and was, strong and consistent evidence for airborne aerosol infection with COVID-19 (Greenhalgh et al. 2024). This is demonstrated and supported, they argue, by the patterning of spread which was mostly indoors, and the high rate of asymptomatic transmission, i.e. occurring when people were not coughing and sneezing.

Greenhalgh and colleagues (2024), (drawing on the research of Darquenne, 2012; Chen et al. 2021; Stadnytskyi et al., 2021 and Bourouiba, 2021) explain why this is.

> Infected individuals, whether symptomatic or not, continuously shed particles containing pathogens, which remain viable for several hours and

> can travel long distances. SARS-CoV-2 is shed mainly from deep in the lungs, not the upper respiratory tract, and the viral load is higher in small aerosols (generated in the lower airways) than in larger droplets (generated in upper airways). Whereas large respiratory droplets emitted when people cough or sneeze fall quickly by force of gravity without much evaporation, those below 100 μm in diameter become (bio)aerosols. Even particles tens of microns in diameter at release will shrink almost immediately by evaporation to the point that under typical conditions they can remain airborne for many minutes. In contrast with droplet transmission, which is generally assumed to occur via a single ballistic hit, the risk of airborne transmission increases incrementally with the amount of time the lung lining is exposed to pathogen-laden air, in other words, with time spent indoors inhaling contaminated air.
>
> *(Greenhalgh et al., 2024: 4)*

Although various authors suggest that airborne transmission is only relevant for 'unusual' diseases, there is in fact robust evidence supporting the airborne transmission of many respiratory viruses, including severe acute respiratory syndrome coronavirus (SARS-CoV), Middle East respiratory syndrome (MERS)–CoV, influenza virus, human rhinovirus, and respiratory syncytial virus (RSV). With COVID-19, the limitations of traditional views of droplet, fomite, and airborne transmission were illuminated as the virus spread. As Wang et al. concluded, 'droplet and fomite transmission of SARS-CoV-2 alone cannot account for the numerous superspreading events and differences in transmission between indoor and outdoor environments observed during the COVID-19 pandemic.' (Wang et al., 2021: 981).

The evidence notwithstanding, from the early months of the pandemic, there were many examples of major health agencies and politicians, including the World Health Organisation promoting what proved to be partial information about how COVID-19 was transmitted and providing misleading instructions as to the best way to prevent the spread – not advocating universal masking and instead focusing on hand and surface hygiene (Greenhalgh et al., 2022). This was reinforced by the publication of the Cochrane Collaboration's review of a synthesis of the evidence from randomised controlled trials of the preventive effectiveness of masks, which was taken to show that mask-wearing was ineffective (Jefferson et al., 2023). The limitations of the Cochrane Review have been widely discussed subsequently, but at the time, the narrative of droplets was reinforced. An early focus on airborne transmission would have led to much greater emphasis on indoor air quality, ventilation, filtration, reducing indoor crowding, and time spent indoors and taking care when speaking, as well as wearing a suitable and effective mask.

While the two modes of transmission are possible, and while preventive measures should have embraced them both, it was the initial preference for the droplet approach which is of interest here. It is so in that the evidence that COVID-19 was airborne was clear, consistent, definitive and largely ignored. Importantly from our perspective sneezing and coughing are intermittent events, whereas breathing and talking are routine normal everyday occurrences embedded in every (in the case of breathing) and very many (in the case of talking) social practices in which humans engage.

In the early days of the pandemic there was much debate about the value of mask-wearing as a consequence of arguments about aerosols and airborne infection. This was complicated by the fact that a mask is not a single thing with a universal design. It is now clear that certain types of masks are much more effective than others. It is now also clear that respirators are significantly more effective than cloth or medical masks. In other words, the evidence has to broaden from a single view about the nature of transmission) (droplets vs aerosols) to a much wider consideration of evidence from indoor ventilation engineering, filtration engineering, the mechanisms of mask manufacture, as well as the everyday activities in which people engage.

This is important in that the initial dominance of the droplet-view meant that measures relating to other theories of contagion were slow to be taken up. Further the droplet approach and the focus on symptomatic people meant that breathing and talking in indoor settings, and the significance of overcrowding in such settings were overlooked or ignored. The instructions to stay home and to not go outside, and the edicts about home working and home education, were likely to have made the situation worse, especially for those for whom crowded home spaces were the norm.

In summary, syndemic interactions involving the virus and its differing modes of transmission, the social conditions in which people live, the ubiquitous presence of virus carrying aerosols and the dynamic social practices of people's lives, were undervalued as a means of explaining both aetiology and prevention. Because the medical model and much public health consistently conflates aetiology and prevention (Kelly and Russo, 2018) – the idea that if you know the cause of a disease you will know what to do to prevent it – meant that in this case because the mainstream aetiological understanding was only partial (i.e. the emphasis on droplets), the preventive measures were also only partial.

A further also significant tendency was to focus on the COVID-19 virus in isolation and to overlook both the social organisation of transmission (of the virus) and the severity, or otherwise, of disease. The effect was to marginalise long standing social and material inequalities, and to position them as additional, but not central, explanations of severe illness or death.

COVID-19 in isolation: Social difference and health

A basic precept of evidence-based medicine (EBM) is to check out what is already known before embarking on new interventions or new research. In the case of COVID-19, this did not happen: instead, well-established connections between social difference and health were simply ignored. This was in spite of the fact that the historical record shows that previous pandemics have had disproportionate impact on the poor and disadvantaged (Bambra et al 2020). There was, in addition, a known interaction between pre-existing medical conditions (often associated with disadvantage) and some coronaviruses (Leung et al., 2004).

Within a few months of the start of lockdown it became clear that there were marked differences between various groups in the British population in terms of the likelihood of serious illness and death as a result of infection. What also became clear was that some ethnic minority groups, some socially disadvantaged populations, older people, and people with pre-existing medical conditions – diabetes, hypertension, cardiovascular disease, chronic obstructive pulmonary disease, chronic kidney disease, obesity, dementia and Alzheimer's disease (Marmot et al., 2020), were at very much higher risk of harm (Bhopal, 2020).

In other words, COVID-19 did not have effects in isolation. Far from being independent of its surroundings, the impact of the disease was mediated by a host of other conditions, including those most strongly associated with health inequalities (Marmot et al., 2020; The Independent Scientific Advisory Group for Emergencies (SAGE) Report, 2020a; 2020b; Public Health England, 2020a; 2020b; Pareek et al., 2020). This is not surprising in that the epigenetic traces of social and biological inheritance, and the effect of previous patterns of diet and exposure on the bodies of people exposed to COVID-19 in the 2020s were well known in the scientific literature. However, they had no role in the policy options being pursued (Barker and Thornburg, 2013; Radford, 2018).

Although the data pointed to a dynamic relation between the virus, pre-existing medical conditions and social circumstances – what has been called a syndemic interaction (Horton, 2020; Singer 2009), careful accounts of these and other such conjunctions were routinely overlooked (Hinchliffe et al., 2021). Despite a twenty-year history in the medical anthropological literature, the syndemic concept was simply not applied to COVID-19 (Horton, 2020; Bambra et al., 2020). This was despite the fact that similar dynamic processes had been identified in the early part of the twentieth century with the outbreaks of SARS (Chan et al., 2003; Chen-Yu et al., 2005; Leung et al., 2004; Wong et al., 2003; Yang et al., 2006).

Interactions between a coronavirus, pre-existing medical conditions and social background had therefore been reported in the mainstream medical literature decades before the COVID-19 pandemic took hold. The evidence that there was a highly predictable effect and that this was a consequence of the intermingling of social practices, was already there in plain sight. Instead of foregrounding what was already known about social differences and health, policies including contact tracing, travel bans, advice not to wear masks and then rules about wearing masks, social gatherings and lockdown, were deployed on the basis of evidence that took little or no account of the uneven effects of past and present practices.

Looking back, patterns of COVID-19 mortality were highly predictable, not because of epidemiological modelling, but on the basis of decades of evidence about co-existing conditions, contagion and social difference, adding up to known patterns of health inequality. Eventually instructions were issued to the NHS to do something about the impact that COVID-19 had on different sectors of the population (Stevens and Pritchard, 2020) but what was to be done remained unspecified. For the most part local jurisdictions simply gathered more data, especially about ethnicity. This was long overdue, for sure, but it was also not something that speeded up responses to the pandemic or made them more effective.

Revisiting COVID-19: Implications for practice theory and public health

In this chapter we have focused on three assumptions underpinning the UK government's response to the COVID-19 pandemic. These include, first, a focus on *individual* behaviour (as if people can choose how they interact, where they go, or how they live); second, a theory of contagion that revolved around the significance of droplets (not aerosols) – hence injunctions to wash hands, clean surfaces and keep 2 metres apart; and third, a persistent tendency to view COVID-19 in isolation, and to focus on the virus as a singular 'entity' the health impact of which was unrelated to co-existing conditions, circumstances and social differences. These are not separate commitments. Rather, they combine and amplify each other as they are reproduced in policy injunctions and responses, and in measures (prior to mass vaccination) to contain the spread of COVID-19 and to manage its impact on the NHS.

Although dominant in policy circles, these positions are at odds with recent social theory, including theories of practice, and with more complex accounts of the relation between biological and medical science and public policy. In what follows we expand on these points of difference, and on the sorts of responses that might have been adopted had politicians and policy makers been willing and able to engage with a wider range of social scientific and medical knowledge, and with what we know about the histories of past practices, interactions and epigenetic processes.

As outlined above, the UK, the government's response to COVID-19 played down the social organisation of daily life, the accumulation of material relations, and the divisions, connections and institutions on which it depends. By contrast, social theorists in general, and practice theorists in particular, suppose that people are the 'carriers' of practices (of ways of living, working and moving around) that exist beyond them, and that extend across space and time (Giddens, 1984). From this, other conclusions follow: current practices bear the traces of the past, as do the material arrangements, and human and non-human bodies associated with them; practices are permeable in the sense that they are not just linked to, but are mutually dependent on and reinforcing of, other practices; and in combination, practices and complexes of them 'prefigure' the future, making some trajectories more likely than others.

By implication, COVID-19 was and is inseparable from these dynamics and from the material arrangements within which the virus circulated and had effect. More specifically, forms of family life, 'events' like Christmas and summer holidays, or football matches proved to be pinch points in efforts to limit social interaction not because they are expressions of individual choice and behaviour but because they are embedded in the flows of practices of which contemporary ways of life are made. Likewise, social divisions and differences do not 'just' occur – they are inscribed in what Bourdieu referred to as the 'habitus' of social life, and in long histories of geographical, temporal and material arrangements, including international travel, house design, methods of ventilating buildings, patterns of employment and more (Bourdieu, 1990).

Crucially, these arrangements vary systematically and in so doing they underpin differences and inequalities, including health inequalities, the risks of exposure, including exposure to viruses like COVID-19, and the likelihood of serious harm. As hinted at above, it would be possible, and feasible, to take this into account and to distinguish between those practices that bring people into close proximity, and those that do not; or to consider the reconfiguring of risk relating to and following from the emergence of 'new' ways of working, for example, working from home, or online. This points towards a more socially informed style of response, not one that supposes that all individuals are equal, or that behavioural change is at heart a matter of individual choice. It also implies a focus on health, rather than on the spread of the virus, as if that was the primary concern.

Understanding how COVID-19 spread, via droplets or aerosols, or some combination of both, brings different sets of practices into view, and by implication, argues for different or multiple forms of intervention relating to quite different sorts of conventions, institutions and material arrangements. To give a couple of examples, shaking hands (or not) involves touch and close proximity, as one hand is pressed against another. But other forms of recognition – including fist bumps – also involve proximity and, as such, make little or no difference to the circulation of virus laden aerosols. If we go along with the aerosol view, it makes sense to focus on matters other than those of greeting, or on the so-called 2 metre rule. Instead, it is ventilation that really counts. This is plainly not a matter of choice in that people live and work in buildings that have air conditioning, or fixed windows, or they are densely packed into small spaces together with family and/or colleagues and in rooms and buildings, the design of which is way beyond their control.

The point is not to conclude that COVID-19 circulates in one way or another, but it is to recognise that alternative theories of infection foreground, or dismiss, different styles and sites of intervention. More than that, it is important to recognise that the scope for intervention differs from case to case, and that in some situations minimising the risk of disease might involve long term modifications to the built environment and the infrastructures that surround us. To put it more concretely, coronaviruses do not spread on their own: they circulate through and because of the relations and materials of the day, and these are, in turn, outcomes and expressions of past and present practices, and of the pathways of actual and potential infection that do and do not arise as a result.

Last, but definitely not least, a more social theoretical approach would, of necessity, focus on relations between practices, and on uneven landscapes of possibility as these are formed by the traces and residues not of one practice at a time, but of entire complexes of them. When seen in this way it makes no sense to focus on COVID-19 as if the virus somehow existed in isolation, or as if its effects were independent of co-existing arrangements, co-morbidities, and the traces and trails (good and bad) of a whole raft of other interdependent practices. More concretely, treating COVID-19 as a virus, separated, isolated and as seen under a microscope or as genetically sequenced, fails to appreciate the ways in which it is intermingled with other social and biological forms, and underplays the ways in which the virus adapts and changes, along with the conditions and circumstances in which it does (or does not) thrive.

Together these few observations hint at the scope for developing and advancing forms of intervention that are compatible with an understanding of how viruses circulate in the world, about how they spread and about how when and where their virulence and toxicity waxes and wanes. They also serve to remind us that although the virus appeared or was recognised apparently quite suddenly, it didn't begin then, in December 2019. Rather than isolating the 'real' origin of coronavirus, the more important insight is that the virus, its impact, and the speed of its circulation, depended on the practices of people, institutions, governments and on the rich mixture of social-biological arrangements which generated susceptibility to infection and established the conditions within and through which the infection spread.

As represented here, the picture is one of a multi-directional flow in which practices affected the virus, and in which the virus also affected the lives of multiple practices, and connections between them. This is not in the least bit unusual. The billions of microbial organisms which inhabit the human body as well as the air and the water and soil in the wider ecology are inseparable from the overlapping lives of multiple practices.

The unequal distribution of these complexes and combinations is important both for patterns of transmission, for the conditions in which COVID-19 had effect, and for the severity of disease. In short, the presence of the virus in aerosols and in droplets meant that in many respects the COVID-19 virus was ubiquitously inescapable, but its capacity to do harm was highly selective, not randomly but on the basis of, and as filtered by, past practices. These are critical insights in that they suggest that to understand the pandemic we must take heed of the criss-crossing of practices in which human and non-human actors are enmeshed, and we must acknowledge the constitution and the shaping of 'biosocial' arrangements, including arrangements in and of which coronavirus is and was a part (Hinchliffe et al., 2021).

This brings us to the vaccine. It is tempting to think of the mass vaccination programme as the end of the story and as a technical fix that undermined the virus and its potential to cause death and serious disease. In many respects that is correct (Hinchliffe et al., 2021). Vaccines saved the day, but a lot of people died, a lot of money was wasted, and a lot of people's lives were turned upside down unnecessarily. In combination, pre- and post-vaccine responses represent moments in a much longer-term relation between people, material environments, viruses and bacteria, all of which are changing all the time.

Rather than separating the social from the biological realm, or the pre and the post vaccine era, our contention is that both are intermingled and that policy responses like those that we have described, including methods of modelling and epidemiology, and injunctions like those of wearing or not wearing masks, keeping two metres apart, and not shaking hands, exist alongside histories of research in microbiology, in pandemic preparedness (in all its forms), and in the globalisation of travel, the circulation of goods, and the very divided economics and politics of trade and employment – all of which depend on a substrate of viral, fungal and microbial life. There are of course different ways of distinguishing between social, biological and physical worlds, and correspondingly different ways of conceptualising either their interaction (for example, Darwin (1859; 1871), Engel (1960), Waddington (1968) and Dubos (1980)), or their inseparable intermingling (Ingold, 2013). What is striking is that during COVID-19, these entangled histories were marginalised in dominant policy responses and analyses in the UK and in other countries besides.

It may be that Anderson (2021) and Kahneman (2011) are right, and that when faced with a global emergency, governments will inevitably fall back on simplistic models and back-of-the-envelope strategies that have little or no connection with what we – and they – know about the world and how it works. But it would be pessimistic to conclude that this is the only option. The current public enquiry into the UK government's response to COVID-19 is of course, framed in its own terms, and is, as such, unlikely to escape the assumptions outlined above.

The pandemic was an emergent property of global intermingling (socially, physically and biologically) which defied simple modelling or simple solutions (Hinchliffe et al., 2021). However, it is possible that future pandemics will be met with a more subtle response, grounded in a more sophisticated understanding of layered and indivisible social, material and biological dynamics, and in correspondingly complex accounts of variation and difference. This would depend on policy processes that are informed by a broad interpretation of scientific evidence, and that incorporate insights from historians and social theorists as well as, or perhaps instead of, epidemiologists and modellers.

This suggests the need for an interpretation of pandemic preparedness that depends on new ways of integrating research and policy. As described above, responses to COVID-19 were founded on a narrow set of guiding assumptions. On reflection, politicians and policy makers did exactly as might be expected, sticking closely to conventional methods of designing and implementing policy, and doing so in times of great uncertainty. In the circumstances it would be unreasonable to expect more, or to imagine that the UK government might have adopted an approach to the problem that took heed of all the 'evidence' at hand, or that took note of the interwoven social histories and processes described above. Equally, and as outlined above, the government's response resulted in far reaching restrictions, a huge loss of life and massive waste.

In this chapter we have deliberately focused on the UK and on responses in England, Wales, Scotland and Northern Ireland. All four jurisdictions pursued similar if not identical policies, and all were based on the sorts of assumptions we have described. We have concentrated on the British experience because it is easy to identify the type of science involved and the principles on which government strategies were based. We are obviously not suggesting that other countries subscribed to the same theories of behaviour, contagion and disease: as we know, efforts to limit the impact of COVID-19 varied depending on the nature of national and local political leadership, cultural and social histories, and structural variations, including the role and influence of public health authorities (Ortega and Orsini, 2020; Milan and Treré, 2020; Power, 2020; Mooi-Reci and Risman, 2021). But as we also know the result, in general, was a failure all round to protect the public, particularly the most vulnerable, to avoid the large numbers of deaths worldwide, and to get to grips with the pandemic in a timely fashion (Meloni and Vatter, 2023: 374).

This lends weight to the suggestion that if they are to avoid repeating the mistakes of the past, policy makers and governments, including the UK government, need to take a broad view of preparedness. In effect preparation for the next pandemic depends on being prepared to take an integrated approach, not as a one-off response, but as a matter of course. This could and should involve the routine adoption of methods of intervening and working that are founded on careful and systemic understanding of the social and geographical ordering of the biosocial flux and of the part that policy does (and does not) play in shaping the multiple dynamics involved.

This might sound like wishful thinking, but there are many examples of subtle and differentiated policies that recognise health inequalities, and the accumulated effects of past practices. Making use of these experiences depends on recognising both the social organisation of transmission and the unequal consequences of infection. In the UK, this rests on a willingness to set limited forms of individualism and epidemiology aside and to acknowledge what we know about the unequal distribution of social practices, and about how these configure also unequal forms of human and non-human interaction. At the end of the day, this is the kind of preparedness that is needed.

References

Anderson, W. (2021). 'The model crisis, or how to have critical promiscuity in the time of Covid-19', *Social Studies of Science,* 51(2): 167–188. https://doi.org/10.1177/0306312721996053.

Bambra C., Riordan, Ryan., Ford, J. and Mathews, F. (2020). 'The COVID-19 pandemic and health inequalities', *Journal of Epidemiology and Community Health*, 74: 964–968. https://doi.org/10.1136/jech-2020-214401.

Barker, D.J.P. and Thornburg, K.L. (2013). 'Placental programming of chronic diseases, cancer and lifespan: A review', *Placenta,* 34: 841–845. http://dx.doi.org/10.1016/j.placenta.2013.07.063

Bhopal, R. (2020). 'Covid-19 worldwide: we need precise data by age group and sex urgently', *British Medical Journal,* 369: m1366 https://doi.org/10.1136/bmj.m1366

Bourdieu, P. (1990). *The Logic of Practice*, Cambridge: Polity.

Bourouiba L. (2021). 'The fluid dynamics of disease transmission', *Annual Review of Fluid Mechanics,* 53: 473–508. https://doi.org/10.1146/annurev-fluid-060220-113712

Box, G. E. P. (1979). 'Robustness in the strategy of scientific model building' in Launer, R. L., and Wilkinson, G. N., (eds.) *Robustness in Statistics*, New York: Academic Press: 201–236.

Chan, J. M.W, Ng, C.K., Chan, Y.H., Mok, T.Y.W., WHO, Lee, S., Chu, S.Y.Y., Law, W.L., Lee, M.P., and Li, P.C. K. (2003). 'Short term outcomes and risk factors for adverse clinical outcomes in adults with severe acute respiratory syndrome', *Thorax,* 58: 686–689. https://thorax.bmj.com/content/thoraxjnl/58/8/686.full.pdf

Chen, P.Z., Bobrovitz, N., Premji, Z., Koopmans, M., Fisman, D.N. and Gu F.X. (2021). 'Heterogeneity in transmissibility and shedding SARS-CoV-2 via droplets and aerosols', *Elife*, https://doi.org/10.7554/eLife.65774.

Chen-Yu, C., Lee, C.H., Liu, C.Y., Wang, J.H., Wang, L.M., Perng, R.P. (2005). 'Clinical features and outcomes of severe acute respiratory syndrome and predictive factors for acute respiratory distress syndrome', *Journal of the Chinese Medical Association*, 68: 4–10. https://doi.og/10.1016/S1726-4901(09)70124-8.

Darquenne C. (2012). 'Aerosol deposition in health and disease', *J Aerosol Med Pulm Drug Deliv*, 25: 140–147. https://doi.org/10.1089/jamp.2011.0916.

Darwin, C. ([1859] 2006). *On the Origin of Species By Means of Natural Selection: Or the Preservation of Favoured Races in the Struggle for Life.* London: Folio.

Darwin, C. ([1871] 1981). *The Descent of Man: And Selection in Relation to Sex.* Princeton, N.J.: Princeton University Press.

Department of Health (2011). 'UK Influenza Pandemic Preparedness Strategy 2011', https://assets.publishing.service.gov.uk/media/5a7c4767e5274a2041cf2ee3/dh_131040.pdf.

Dubos, R. (1980). *Man Adapting.* New Haven: Yale University Press.

Engel, G.L. (1960). 'A unified concept of health and disease', *Perspectives in Biology and Medicine*, 3: 459–485.

Giddens, A. (1984). *The Constitution of Society: Outline of the theory of structuration.* Cambridge: Polity.

Greenhalgh, T., MacIntyre, C.R., Baker, M.G., Bhattacharjee, S., Chughtai, A.A., Fisman, D., Kunasekaran, M., Kvalsvig, A., Lupton, D., Oliver, M., Tawfiq, E., Ungrin, M. and Vipond, J. (2024). 'Masks and respirators for prevention of respiratory infections: a state of the science review', *Clinical Microbiology Reviews,* 37(2): 1–63. https://doi.org/10.1128/cmr.00124-23.

Greenhalgh, T., Ozbilgin, M., and Tomlinson, D. (2022). 'How covid-19 spreads: narratives, counter narratives, and social dramas', *British Medical Journal*, 378: e069940. https://doi.org/10.1136/bmj-2022-069940

Hallett H. (2024). *UK Covid-19 Inquiry Module 1: The Resilience and Preparedness of the United Kingdom.* https://covid19.public-inquiry.uk/documents/module-1-full-report/. London, UK: HMSO.

Hinchliffe S., Manderson L., and Moore, M. (2021). 'Planetary healthy publics after COVID-19', *Lancet Planet Health,* 5: e230–e236. Available at: www.thelancet.com/action/showPdf?pii=S2542-5196%2821%2900050-4.

Horton, R. (2020). 'Offline: COVID-19 is not a pandemic', *Lancet*, 396: 874, 26 September 2020. www.thelancet.com/action/showPdf?pii=S0140-6736%2820%2932000-6.

Ingold, T. (2013). 'Prospect' in Ingold, T. and Pálsson, G. (eds.) *Biosocial Becomings: Integrating social and biological anthropology.* Cambridge: Cambridge University Press: 1–21. https://doi.org/10.1017/CBO9781139198394.

Jefferson, T., Dooley, L., Ferroni, E., Al-Ansary L.A., van Driel, M.L., Bawazeer, G.A., Jones, M.A., Hoffmann, T.C., Clark, J., Beller, E.M., Glasziou, P.P., and Conly, J.M. (2023). 'Physical interventions to interrupt or reduce the spread of respiratory viruses', *Cochrane Database Syst Rev*, 1. https://doi.org/10.1002/14651858.CD006207.pub5

Kahneman, D. (2011). *Thinking, Fast and Slow*. New York: Farrar, Strauss and Giroux.

Kelly, M.P. (2021). 'Ontological uncertainty and ontological threat: COVID-19 and the UK', *Perspectives in Biology and Medicine*, 64(3): 316–337. https://doi.org/10.1353/pbm.2021.0024.

Kelly, M.P. and Barker, M. (2016). 'Why is changing health related behaviour so difficult?', *Public Health*, 136: 109–116. https://doi.org/10.1016/j.puhe.2016.03.030

Kelly, M.P. and Russo, F. (2018). 'Causal narratives in public health: the difference between mechanisms of aetiology and mechanisms of prevention in non-communicable diseases', *Sociology of Health and Illness*, 40(1): 82–99. https://doi.org/10.1111/1467-9566.12621/pdf

Kelly, M.P. and Russo, F. (2021). 'The epistemic values at the basis of epidemiology and public health', *Mefisto*, 5(1): 105–120. https://doi.org/10.4454/mefisto.5-1.

Kucharski, A. J., Russell, T.W., Diamond, C., Liu, Y., Edmunds, J., Funk, S. and Eggo, R.M. (2020). 'Early dynamics of transmission and control of COVID-19: a mathematical modelling study', *Lancet Infectious Diseases,* 20(5): 553–558. https://doi.org/10.1016/S1473-3099(20)30144-4.

Laing, R.D. (1976). *The Politics of the Family and Other Essays*. Harmondsworth: Pelican Books.

Leung, G.M., Hedley, A.J., Ho, L-M., Chau, P., Wong, I.O.L., Thach, T.Q., Ghani, A.C., Donnelly, C.A., Fraser, C., Riley, S., Ferguson, N.M., Anderson, R.M., Tsang, T., Leung, P-Y., Wong, V., Chan, J.C.K., Tsui, E., Lo, S.V. and Lam, T.H., (2004). 'The epidemiology of severe acute respiratory syndrome in the 2003 Hong Kong epidemic: An analysis of all 1755 patients', *Annals of Internal Medicine*, 141: 662–673. https://doi.org/10.7326/0003-4819-141-9-200411020-00006.

Marmot, M., Allen, J., Goldblatt, P., Herd, E. and Morrison, J. (2020). 'Build Back Fairer: The COVID-19 Marmot Review: The Pandemic, Socioeconomic and Health Inequalities in England'. London: Institute of Health Equity. www.instituteofhealthequity.org/resources-reports/build-back-fairer-the-covid-19-marmot-review/build-back-fairer-the-covid-19-marmot-review-full-report.pdf

Marres, N. and Valderrama Barragán, M. (2025). 'Making expert advice public in a time of emergency: Independent SAGE and the contestation of science during the Covid pandemic in the UK', *Social Studies of Science,* 55(4): 512–541. https://doi.org/10.1177/03063127241309071

Marteau, T. M., Ogilvie, D., Roland, M., Suhrcke, M., and Kelly, M.P. (2011). 'Judging nudging: can "nudging" improve population health?', *British Medical Journal,* 342: d228. https://doi.org/10.1136/bmj.d228.

Meloni, M. and Vatter, M. (2023). 'Biopolitics After COVID: Notes from the Crisis', *Theory and Event*, 26(2): 368–392. https://doi.org/10.1353/tae.2023.0019.

Milan, S. and Treré, E. (2020). 'The Rise of the Data Poor: The COVID-19 Pandemic Seen from the Margins', *Social Media and Society*, 6(3): 1–8. https://doi.org/10.1177/2056305120948233.

Mooi-Reci I., and Risman, B.J. (2021). 'The gendered impacts of COVID-19: Lessons and reflections', *Gender and Society,* 35(2):161–167. https://doi.org/10.1177/08912432211001305.

Ortega, F. and Orsini, M. (2020). 'Governing COVID-19 without government in Brazil: Ignorance, neoliberal authoritarianism, and the collapse of public health leadership', *Global Public Health,* 15(9): 1257–1277. https://doi.org/10.1080/17441692.2020.1795223.

Pareek, M., Bangash, M.N., Pareek, N., Pan, D., Sze, S., Minhas, J.S., Hanif, W. and Khunti, K. (2020). 'Ethnicity and COVID-19: an urgent public health research priority', *Lancet,* 395: 1421–1422. https://doi.org/10.1016/S0140-6736(20)30922-3.

Power, K. (2020). 'The COVID-19 pandemic has increased the care burden of women and families', *Sustainability: Science, Practice and Policy,* 16(1): 67–73. https://doi.org/10.1080/15487733.2020.1776561.

Public Health England (2020a). *Disparities in the risk and outcomes of COVID-19.* Public Health England: London. https://assets.publishing.service.gov.uk/government/uploads/system/uploads/attachment_data/file/908434/Disparities_in_the_risk_and_outcomes_of_COVID_August_2020_update.pdf

Public Health England (2020b). *Beyond the data: Understanding the impact of COVID-19 on BAME groups.* London: Public Health England. https://assets.publishing.service.gov.uk/government/uploads/system/uploads/attachment_data/file/892376/COVID_stakeholder_engagement_synthesis_beyond_the_data.pdf.

Radford, E. (2018). 'Exploring the extent and scope of epigenetic inheritance', *Nature Reviews Endocrinology,* 14: 345–355. https://doi.org/10.1038/s41574-018-0005-5.

Russo, F. and Kelly, M.P. (2023). 'The "lifeworld" of health and disease and the design of public health interventions', *Longitudinal and Life Course Studies,* 15(1): 25–44. https://doi.org/10.1332/175795921X16835353334712.

Russo, F. and Williamson, J. (2007). 'Interpreting causality in the health sciences', *International Studies in Philosophy of Science,* 21(2): 157–170. https://doi.org/10.1080/02698590701498084

Russo, F. and Williamson J. (2011). 'Epistemic causality and evidence-based medicine', *History and Philosophy of the Life Sciences,* 33: 563–582. Available at: https://pubmed.ncbi.nlm.nih.gov/22662510/.

Shove, E., Blue, S., and Kelly, M.P. (2026). *Practice Theory and the Biosocial: Microbes, matter and milieu.* Oxford: Berghahn Books. https://doi.org/10.3167/9781836953395.

Singer, M. (2009). *Introduction to Syndemics: A Critical Systems Approach to Public and Community Health.* San Francisco: Jossey-Bass.

Stadnytskyi V., Anfinrud P. and Bax A. (2021). 'Breathing, speaking, coughing or sneezing: what drives transmission of SARS-CoV-2?', *J Intern Med,* 290: 1010–1027. https://doi.org/10.1111/joim.13326.

Stevens, S. and Pritchard, A. (2020). 'Letter to Trusts, CCGs, Primary Care, Community Health Service Providers, NHS111, 31st July 2020'. Available at: www.england.nhs.uk/coronavirus/wp-content/uploads/sites/52/2020/07/20200731-Phase-3-letter-final-1.pdf.

The Independent Scientific Advisory Group for Emergencies (SAGE) (2020a). *Disparities in the impact of COVID-19 in Black and Minority Ethnic populations: review of the evidence and recommendations for action, The Independent SAGE Report 6.* Available at: www.independentsage.org/wp-content/uploads/2020/07/Independent-SAGE-BME-Report_02July_FINAL.pdf

The Independent Scientific Advisory Group for Emergencies (SAGE) (2020b). *COVID-19 and Health Inequality. The Independent SAGE Report 21.* Available at: www.independentsage.org/wp-content/uploads/2020/11/Inequalities-_i_SAGE_FINAL-draft_corrected.pdf

Waddington, C. H. (1968). 'The basic ideas of biology' in Waddington, C. H. (ed) *Towards a Theoretical Biology*, Volume 1. Edinburgh: Edinburgh University Press: 1–32.

Wang, C.C., Prather, K. A., Sznitman, J., Jimenez, J. L., Lakdawala, S.S., Tufekci, Z., Marr, L.C. (2021). 'Airborne transmission of respiratory viruses', *Science,* 373, eabd9149. https://doi.org/10.1126/science.abd9149.

Wong, W-W., Chen, T-L., Yang, S-P., Wang, F-D., Cheng, N.C., Ing-Tiau Kuo, B., Yu, K-W., Tsai, C-A., Lin, Y-S., Lee, I-R., Chi, C-Y., Lai, C-J., Lai, C-H., Chen, H-P. and Liu, C-Y. (2003). 'Clinical characteristics of fatal patients with severe acute respiratory syndrome in a medical centre in Taipei', *Journal of the Chinese Medical Association*, 66(6): 323–327. Available at: https://pubmed.ncbi.nlm.nih.gov/12889500/.

Yang, J. K., Feng, Y., Yuan, M.Y., Yuan, S.Y., Fu, H.J., Wu, B.Y., Sun, G.Z., Yang, G.R., Zhang, X.L., Wang, L., Xu, X., Xu, X.P. and Chan, J.C.N. (2006). 'Plasma glucose levels and diabetes are independent predictors for mortality and morbidity in patients with SARS', *Diabetic Medicine,* 23: 623–628. https://doi.org/10.1111/j.1464-5491.2006.01861.x

12

WHAT PRACTICE THEORIES BRING TO STUDIES OF MICROBES AND SOCIETIES

Elizabeth Shove, Cecily Maller and Simon Cohn

Introduction

We began by promising a book that would challenge established ideas about microbes and societies, and about bodies, diseases and health. In this last chapter we revisit that promise, taking stock of what has been achieved and what remains to be done. We do so by means of a dialogue between two imaginary readers: Angela (Reader A), who concludes that we *augment* existing schools of thought and Barbara (Reader B), who contends that we *upend* those same traditions.

Both fictional readers agree that this book rejects dominant ways of thinking about human-microbial relations, both go along with the view that the planet is inhabited and constituted by multitudes of bacteria, viruses and microbial entities and both are interested in what social theories mean for the study of microscopic matter. However, their responses reveal significantly different ideas about what this entails.

In mapping out contrasting interpretations of the chapters included in this collection, we start with the suggestion that the social organisation of practices is important for when and where people and microbes meet.

Encounters or configurations

Angela is the first to comment.

> Epidemiologists tend to describe the geographies of infection as outcomes of social conditions, but other traditions, including feminism and actor network theory, take a broader view of when, where and how people

DOI: 10.4324/9781003685210-16

> and microbes meet, for good or ill. This is a useful and interesting book because it adds to this literature and brings a practice lens to bear on pro- and antibiotic encounters in farms, homes, school playgrounds, parks, hospitals and more.
>
> *(Anglea)*

Barbara responds.

> I agree this is an important collection, but in my opinion, it is so because it *resists* the concepts and traditions to which you refer. It is true that some contributors treat human and more-than-human encounters as effects of social practice, but I prefer the more radical conclusion that people and microbes change *together*, as practices and complexes of them evolve and combine. In my view, understanding contagion is a matter of understanding situated configurations of practice, *not* of describing patterns of human exposure to benign and/or pathogenic microbes.
>
> *(Barbara)*

This might seem like a matter of emphasis – some contributors describe human-microbial encounters, and some write about the changing geometries of intermingling – but for Angela and Barbara these approaches depend on fundamentally different interpretations of practice theory and of what it has to offer.

Microscopic materials and practices

As is always the case, questions and lines of enquiry are defined by prior theoretical commitments. By way of illustration, Angela is interested in how human and more-than-human entities intra-act in a given context, and in what this means for patterns of health and/or disease. She is consequently in favour of multispecies analyses and of relational approaches that show how networks of people and microscopic matter take the form they do. Having read this book she is convinced that practice theories can make a useful contribution to this agenda.

By contrast, Barbara believes that social practices, distributed across space and time, represent both the site and the medium of co-constitutive processes in which the 'bio' and the 'social' are inextricably entangled. She is interested in how practices are carried and transformed by people and by microbes alike, and she is excited by the novelty of studies that focus on these dynamics.

While Angela scours the pages for insights into how humans and more-than-humans shape each other (for good or ill), Barbara works through the same chapters in the hope of learning about material flows and processes of becoming.

The porosity of bodies: Implications for practice theory

It is widely accepted that bodies are permeable and mutable in the moment, as nutrients and toxins circulate across boundaries, and in epigenetic processes that occur over the longer run. Angela, who is already convinced that situations and events involve combinations of human and more-than-human beings, is not troubled by this idea. But for Barbara, the porosity of bodies, and especially human bodies, is a more complex topic. Amongst other things, she is intrigued by the claim that people represent the crossing points of processes that run through them and beyond them.

> This way of thinking generates lines of enquiry that are not at all the same as those that show how multiple boundaries co-exist and shape each other. In my view, the refusal to treat human bodies as bounded entities is as unsettling for actor network theory as it is for other traditions in the social and natural sciences. Some contributors give a sense of the turmoil that ensues, but this is just the start. Who knows where analyses of flow and metabolisation might lead, or what new challenges might arise.
>
> *(Barbara)*

In effect, Angela treats human and more-than-human beings as sites in which cells, bacteria, viruses and fungi converge. By contrast, Barbara takes bodies to be more fluid and also more amorphous vessels through which microscopic materials pass. Other differences follow, including Angela's tendency to focus on specific moments in time and space, and Barbara's interest in longer-term histories and processes of change.

Discourses, practices and the politics of knowledge

Existing paradigms matter for how the chapters in this book are read, and for the inspiration they provide. For example, Angela and Barbara agree that ideas about human and planetary health, well-being and risk are reproduced in the details of everyday and professional life, and in policy interventions, past and present. However, they disagree about how these relations should be conceptualised and understood. This is important for the questions on which they focus and for what they overlook.

For Angela, and for others like her, it is important to uncover the hidden politics of dominant narratives and discourses. She elaborates on this theme:

> As Latour pointed out, quite some years ago, theories – in his case about germs – transformed hospitals and hospital life and created dangers where none existed before. In describing the persistent influence of notions of 'balance' and the ideological foundation of epidemiological 'evidence',

> contributors to this book reveal the performative effects of the terms in which problems are framed. To my mind, this is another useful and important contribution.
>
> *(Angela)*

Barbara concurs but she wants to understand *how* theories are woven into complexes of practices including those of research, care, agriculture, medicine and policy intervention.

> Latour's work on the Pasteurization of France is impressive, but it leaves lots of questions unanswered, including questions about how paradigms based on humors or on germs bridge between different areas of daily life, how they become dominant and how they change. What is missing, but what this book provides, is a reminder of how interlocking configurations of practice set the scene for what happens next. As responses to COVID-19 demonstrate, dominant paradigms of individualism infuse ordinary and extreme moments of intervention and legitimise policies (such as lockdown) that are designed to apply equally to all sectors of society. This is just one example, but it points to the inseparability of discourses and material arrangements, and it forces us to think about how specific combinations take the form they do.
>
> *(Barbara)*

This exchange touches on a much bigger debate about the status of concepts like power and inequality, aspects of which are inscribed in the preceding chapters. If you work back through the contributions included in this collection, you will discover that these terms are mobilised in very different ways. In brief, some take power and inequality to be factors that explain the distribution of social practices whereas others conclude that differences (and similarities) are *outcomes* of the interwoven lives of practices and related patterns of accumulation, as these evolve over time.

There is always more to say, and there are always more threads to follow, but it is time to bring this discussion to a close, and to ask Angela and Barbara for a few words about the relevance of this book and the impact it might have on policy makers charged with the task of combatting threats from viruses, allergens, antimicrobial resistance and the spread of infection.

Relevance and impact

Again, Angela is first off the mark.

> I like this collection because it contributes to a growing body of research that documents the interplay of biological, social and material factors. At

> a minimum, policy makers need to recognise that infrastructures, systems of provision and dominant discourses are involved in making patterns of microbial exposure what they are today.
>
> *(Angela)*

Barbara is also positive, but for her the contribution is more profound.

> This book represents a seismic shift in the theoretical foundations of the social and natural sciences. It does so in that taking practices (which are simultaneously human and more-than-human) to be the central topics of conceptualisation and analysis runs counter to more familiar positions in biology, anthropology, geography and sociology. (Barbara)

For Barbara, the answer to the 'so what' question relates to the potential for overhauling mainstream agendas in research and policy. The methodological strategy of focusing on practices, above all, is not without its problems: researchers have to define the always fluid margins of 'a' practice and they need ways of describing changing bundles of practices as these evolve over time. But the promise, and the prize is to grasp, and in fact foreground, forms of flow (of bodies, pathogens, 'good' microbes, nutrients, toxins) that elude other intellectual traditions.

This gestalt switch argues for more historical analyses of how complexes of practices arise and for greater emphasis on related processes including those of metabolic transformation. Finally, and for those involved in policy making, this move positions government policies and international relations and regulations *within* and not outside the intermingling of human and more-than-human life.

Angela and Barbara are invented characters, but their responses suggest that this book is likely to be interpreted in very different ways. This is not just because people bring their own ideas to bear on what they read. That is always so. But it is also not the whole story. In this case, readers of all persuasions are confronted by a text that points in different directions at once.

To put it bluntly, the chapters in this collection do not represent a seamless narrative told from a single point of view. Instead, the seemingly shared language of practice disguises rifts of theory and method that cut through the text as a whole. This is not a problem, nor is it a surprise. After all, chapters are written by authors who come from an impressively diverse mixture of disciplines and traditions, and who develop subtly and sometimes strongly divergent positions on the question of what practice theories bring to the study of microscopic matter.

The overall effect is necessarily unpredictable, but it is through juxtapositions like these that new ideas arise and fresh challenges emerge.

This is just as well. It is true that the future is unknown, but as we explained in the introduction, globally significant problems, including antimicrobial resistance and future pandemics, arise not on their own but from the interweaving of microbes within and as part of society.

INDEX

Note: Tables are indicated by **bold**.

For Product Safety Concerns and Information please contact our EU
representative GPSR@taylorandfrancis.com
Taylor & Francis Verlag GmbH, Kaufingerstraße 24, 80331 München, Germany

www.ingramcontent.com/pod-product-compliance
Ingram Content Group UK Ltd.
Pitfield, Milton Keynes, MK11 3LW, UK
UKHW020007200926
475702UK00015B/2524
* 9 7 8 1 0 4 1 1 6 5 5 6 9 *